WHEN A DOCTOR
HATES A PATIENT

WHEN A DOCTOR HATES A PATIENT
and other chapters in a young physician's life

Richard E. Peschel
and
Enid Rhodes Peschel

UNIVERSITY OF CALIFORNIA PRESS

Berkeley Los Angeles London

University of California Press
Berkeley and Los Angeles, California

University of California Press, Ltd.
London, England

Library of Congress Cataloging-in-Publication Data
Peschel, Richard E.
   When a doctor hates a patient
   Bibliography: p.
   1. Physicians—Training of.   2. Medicine—Case
studies.   3. Humanistic psychology.   4. Medicine in
literature.   I. Peschel, Enid Rhodes.   II. Title.
[DNLM: 1. Internship and Residency—personal narratives.
2. Medicine in Literature.   3. Physicians—personal
narratives.   WZ 100 P473]
R737.P42137   1986   610'.7'11   85-23225
ISBN 0-520-05755-4 (alk. paper)

1 2 3 4 5 6 7 8 9

This book is dedicated to all those involved in
the human experience of medicine

CONTENTS

PREFACE

A note on who we are and how we came to write this book might be helpful. Richard E. Peschel, M.D., Ph.D., is Associate Professor of Therapeutic Radiology and Director of the Residency Program in Therapeutic Radiology at Yale University School of Medicine. Enid Rhodes Peschel, Ph.D., is Co-Director (with Howard Spiro, M.D.) of the Program for Humanities in Medicine at Yale University School of Medicine. A literary scholar and poet-translator, she has published several books, including *Medicine and Literature*.[1]

When *Medicine and Literature* was published in 1980, we were already working on this book. We had begun it in 1977–78, when Richard Peschel was a medical intern. He would come home from the hospital and tell Enid about some of the cases he had treated—those that particularly interested or troubled him—and sometimes Enid would say, "That reminds me of something I read in literature." After a while, we actively sought parallels between real medical case histories and passages in literature. We found that through these parallels we could begin to come to terms with some of the experiences Richard Peschel was living through as a doctor; for literature, which offers a reflection of and on life, sheds light on medicine in that it can serve as the bridge between intense medical experience and all human experience. Because great writers probe life from deeper perspectives and with greater clarity than the ordinary person, one may gain new understanding of the medical experience by pairing real medical case histories with depictions in literature of similar or related problems or themes. By linking the medical experience in literature with their own personal experiences as physicians, many doctors may find comfort and a new understanding of their own fears, hatreds, and limitations.

Because all of our case histories come from Richard Peschel's early encounters in medicine—his years of medical school, internship, and residency—we have called these experiences "chapters in a young physician's life," stressing the relative newness and freshness of the doctor's experiences, impressions, and reactions. During his first years, many things still startle the doctor-in-training and the young doctor. He may react emotionally to events that in later years—when he has witnessed many similar events—become less shocking and even routine to him. In many ways, the new doctor's reactions are different from those of a clinician who has been practicing medicine for some twenty or thirty years. Still, the young doctor's responses undoubtedly evoke resonances with the seasoned practitioner's life. We offer these case histories, literary parallels, and reflections for what they are: the impressions and reactions of a relatively new doctor and our joint effort to try to comprehend and come to terms with the rich—often shocking, unsettling, and frightening, sometimes uplifting, and always astonishing—human experience that is medicine.

ACKNOWLEDGMENTS

For the many valuable suggestions they made as we were working on this book, we wish to express our deepest gratitude to Staige D. Blackford, Diana Festa-McCormick, Robert J. Glaser, M.D., Helen H. Glaser, M.D., Laurence Goldstein, Raymond C. La Charité, Paul E. Molumphy, M.D., Henri Peyre, Sharon Romm, M.D., Nathan N. Rosen, and Richard Selzer, M.D. We also wish to thank Bettyann Kevles, our editor at the University of California Press, for her enthusiasm, support, and very sensitive and helpful advice.

Some chapters of this book first appeared in somewhat different form in the following journals: chapter 2, "My Cadaver: Case History, Literary Histories," *Medical Heritage,* in press; chapter 3, " 'But What If She Should Die?'—Case Histories, Literary Histories—A Discussion of Maternal Death in Childbirth," *The Pharos* 44, no. 1 (Winter 1981); chapter 4, "Ritual and the Death Certificate: Case Histories, Literary Histories," *The Pharos* 46, no. 2 (Spring 1983); chapter 5, "The Tubercular Patient in Art and in Life: Literary History, Case History," *Medical Heritage* 1, no. 6 (Nov.–Dec. 1985); chapter 6, "Aberrant Medical Humor: Case Histories, Literary Histories," *The Pharos* 48, no. 1 (Winter 1985); chapter 7, "When a Doctor Hates a Patient: Case History, Literary Histories," *Michigan Quarterly Review* XXIII, no. 3 (Summer 1984); chapter 9, " 'Am I in Heaven Now?': Case History, Literary Histories," *Soundings* LXVI, no. 4 (Winter 1983); chapter 10, "The Survivor: Case History, Literary Histories," *Medical Heritage* 1, no. 1 (Jan.–Feb. 1985).

INTRODUCTION

Medical training, which includes four years of medical school, one year of internship, plus three or more years of residency, stands apart from ordinary human experience in much the same way that war lies outside the normal realm. Medical training, like combat, involves extraordinary encounters and practices.

Three factors in particular help explain why medical training differs so much from ordinary life. First, the *intensity* of emotion, work load, responsibility, and knowledge required is beyond the average. Very few people have to remember as many facts, work as many hours, read and absorb as many pages, interact with as many emotionally distraught people, and take care of as many persons as do doctors-in-training. Second, the *stakes* involved in medicine are extraordinarily high. Life itself is the currency of medicine, much as it is in war. Mistakes by physicians are costly in terms of suffering and death. Finally, very few other human activities involve such *immersion in death*. One need only see a first-year anatomy class dissecting cadavers to appreciate how early the death immersion process begins.

Unfortunately, because of the enormous pressure of work to be done, the material to be absorbed, and the sophisticated scientific method required to master modern medicine, few students of medicine become students of the emotional, human, and humane aspects of medicine. Most doctors instead are trained to subvert, deflect, or bury their true feelings and reactions and to intellectualize their patients' sufferings and deaths. This intellectualizing is a necessary process toward the rational and scientific treatment of disease, but there is more to medicine than the merely rational and scientific. We believe that doctors can become better healers when they recognize their own human reactions to death and suffering during their training—and afterwards.

Certainly, we are not the only ones to believe this. In recent years, numerous medical educators have recognized and even championed the importance of the human in medicine. Their recognition is evident in the relatively new and expanding field of medicine and literature or, in a broader sense, medicine and the humanities. Many medical schools now offer formal elective courses in medicine and literature or courses that relate medicine to other aspects of the humanities, including philosophy and ethics. There are several explanations for this.

There is, at present, a growing dissatisfaction with medical school curricula. The four years of medical school and the years of internship, residency, and, often, two or more years of a specialty fellowship that follow emphasize the sophisticated, technical aspects of medicine to the virtual exclusion of the humane elements. Whereas medical students are carefully trained in such areas as biochemistry, pathology, laboratory medicine, anatomy, and physical diagnosis, as well as in the latest innovations of life-monitoring and life-supporting gadgetry, they are seldom exposed—if they are exposed at all—to the thought processes necessary for evaluating, understanding, and appreciating what it means to be a patient who is sick, in pain, terrified, or dying. This emphasis on the technological has contributed to the dehumanization of modern medicine. The new doctor is well trained to take care of a body but not of a person. We wish to stress that it is not the emphasis on the scientific, technological, and quantifiable that is to blame for the dehumanization of modern medicine: it is the emphasis on these at the expense of the human that is so unfortunate. And when medical care is dehumanized, both the patient and the physician are losers.

The dehumanizing process of medical education actually begins early in college, where future medical students often adhere to the premedical track with its heavy emphasis on courses in the sciences. Of course, these science requirements are set by the medical schools, and it is obvious that a grounding in science is necessary for a modern medical education. But while medical school admissions committees generally demand that their applicants present outstanding achievements in science, they generally deemphasize equally outstanding backgrounds—suggesting different but equally outstanding abilities—in humanities and arts. The result is that our medical schools are full of superbly trained, sophisticated technicians in the medical sciences who often have an excessively narrow humanistic background on which to draw to broaden and deepen their thought processes.

A related outcome of this selection process is that many people trained as bright, innovative thinkers, including writers, musicians, artists, philosophers, language experts, historians, and students of literature, have been systematically excluded from medicine. Some of those with expertise in the humanities and the arts could easily adjust to a rigorous science program once in medical school. Education in the sciences teaches a person to think in one way; education in the humanities and the arts teaches one to think and to approach problems in other ways. Medicine, which intimately involves both science and the human being, could profit from diverse ways of thinking and solving problems.

Another shortcoming of medical education is that medical students and physicians have little exposure to language at its best, that is, the language of great literature. Premedical students, medical students, and practicing physicians read countless scientific articles detailing the latest research in the basic sciences and medicine. But all these scientific articles are written in the worst style imaginable: the dehumanized, passive, so-called objective style mandated by modern scientific journals. This language—rather, this misuse, mutilation, and murdering of language—purports to be nonpersonal and therefore scientific. In fact, it is dehumanized, dead, and deadening. It dulls the senses and the mind. The jargon of contemporary scientific journals is not an acceptable model for effective communication. Yet this is the language model on which doctors are nurtured, trained, and sustained.

Medicine, however, is not lifeless: it treats the stuff of life. Physicians could profit from intense exposure to the colorful, rich, feeling, expressive, and probing language of literature. The fine use, tuning, and understanding of language are crucial to meaningful human communication. And is not one of the most meaning-charged communications the interchange, precisely, that occurs between a patient and the physician tending him? Perhaps if physicians could learn to express themselves better, to listen to their patients better, to understand what their patients are implying by their words, tones, and gestures, they might be able to communicate more effectively with them. In his introduction to _Medicine and Literature,_ Edmund D. Pellegrino, M.D., one of the pioneers in the field of medicine and the humanities, stresses the importance of language—and therefore of literature—to the physician, since one of the physician's primary jobs is to listen and communicate.

> Literature . . . teaches the physician something of the significance of symbol and language as the media linking human minds and personalities. Language is the instrument of diagnosis and therapy, the vehicle through which the patient's needs are expressed and the doctor's advice conveyed. Understanding the nuances of language, its cultural and ethnic variations and its symbolic content are as essential as any skills the clinician may possess.[1]

Yet another reason that literature, language, and other humanistic studies are being recognized as relevant to medical studies is that a technological explosion has occurred in medicine which has created new ethical dilemmas: terminally ill patients can now be kept artificially alive on life-support systems well beyond their natural lives; artificial hearts can replace a patient's damaged heart; amniocentesis can detect potential birth defects prior to birth; genetic engineering brings an entirely new horizon of scientific intervention. All of these advances raise questions that cut across medical, religious, ethical, philosophical, and societal boundaries. As the chief engineers and representatives of the medical profession, physicians are forced to participate actively in finding solutions to these new ethical dilemmas. Yet, by training, most physicians have little or no special background to help them deal with such profound problems of a multidisciplinary nature.

A very distressing problem today is an outgrowth of the technological explosion. A large proportion of practicing physicians suffer a kind of technological isolation in their practice of medicine. They tend to divorce their daily handling of life, death, and health issues from the larger context of human experience in general. This technological isolation is detrimental both to the physician and to the patient. To some extent, of course, the physician must be objective and unemotional, distanced from his patient and from his patient's suffering, so that he may make a rational judgment about the best treatment to recommend. Still, the doctor must be able to understand and relate to his patient as a thinking, feeling human being.

Although the physician's technological isolation may be seen as a result of his highly technical, essentially nonhumanistic training, it may also be seen as one of his defenses: a shield that protects him from his patient's suffering and pain. But the doctor's isolation is also his burden; it prevents him from reaching out to his patient, and it inhibits him from broadening and deepening his own emotional world, which is, in fact, not so different from his patient's emotional world. After all, what doctor does not become, at some time, a patient? And what doctor, like his patient, is not plagued, at some time, by haunting fears, worries, doubts, and feelings of sadness?

For all the above reasons, and more, it has been recognized that something is missing in the training and education of the modern physician. The discipline of medicine and literature, or medicine and the humanities, is emerging to try to help fill that vacuum. This work is an attempt to contribute to this humanistic movement in medicine.

Each chapter of our book contains one or more medical case histories from Richard Peschel's experience. Since each case history relates a very personal experience, all are told in the first person, the "I" being, of course, Richard Peschel. Even though all the patients in the case histories have passed away, all names and other identifying details have been changed to protect everyone's privacy. In every chapter, the case histories are accompanied by literary parallels, examples from literature which treat similar or related themes or ideas. The literary parallels were chosen by Enid Peschel. Each chapter concludes with a discussion of how the literary parallels illuminate and amplify the medical case or cases. Because these discussions summarize the reflections of both of us, we have deliberately used the plural "we."

Our literary selections come from a wide variety of epochs and cultures, from the ancient Greeks to modern times. We did this because we did not want to limit ourselves to a single era, country, or culture. Instead, we wanted to sound something of the human experience common to all men which cuts across time, space, language, and land. One of our primary aims is to illustrate, through many varied examples, how great literature can help physicians, other health care professionals, and lay persons understand something about the human dramas and dilemmas of medical life. We also hope that the literary examples we use will encourage our readers, medical and nonmedical alike, to look further to literature for many more insights into medicine, man, and life itself.

Starting from the rich human drama—people in moments of crisis, in pain, filled with fear—that a doctor not only witnesses but in which he also participates (sometimes playing a crucial part), we go on to explore, through examples from literature, what other people have done or thought in similar circumstances. Literature offers a wealth of information about how human beings think, feel, act and react, speak and/or are silent. In his daily work, the physician may see or experience some of these feelings and reactions both in his patients and in himself, but he may not be able to probe or explore them much deeper on his own. The literary parallels we use may permit the reader to stand back and watch those feelings and events, think about them, judge them, and try to understand and come to terms with them.

We recognize that our book emphasizes the doctor's role. This, of course, is but one aspect of the total medical picture, only one type of interaction that occurs between a patient and health care professionals. Nurses, medical technologists, receptionists, nurses' aides, physicians' associates, and orderlies make an enormous contribution to the care of patients, and they all have their own unique relationships with patients. Although their interactions with patients may differ in detail from the doctor's, their experiences are similar to his because all involve intimate, human contact with people who are often in pain, frightened, and feeling terribly alone. And so, although our book gives just the physician's viewpoint, we believe it will appeal to numerous other health care professionals who have had countless similar experiences in medicine. Rather than suggesting that the experiences and feelings in our book are unique to physicians, we wish to emphasize that they are common to all of medicine.

We try here to relate one doctor's modest experience and to find for it parallels in human experience portrayed in what Virginia Woolf called "that complete statement which is literature."[2] The medical case histories related here actually took place. Although some of them may seem bizarre, shocking, or unbelievable, they in fact reflect aspects of the common medical experience. Other doctors and health care professionals could tell similar tales, strange in the same ways or in different ways but all suggesting the strengths and weaknesses, fine points and limitations, victories and defenses of the baffled and baffling creature called man.

We hope this marriage between medicine and literature will give the public a greater understanding of the doctor of modern medicine. We also hope these case histories and literary parallels will give the practicing physician a greater insight into himself. We would be glad if our book inspired others—doctors, other health care professionals, patients, and relatives and friends of patients—to probe, judge, and question some of the human and medical events through which they have lived. We know that these chapters from a young doctor's life, along with the literary parallels and our joint reflections, are but a small sampling of what is, in reality, the vast, vital, intense—and moving—human experience of medicine.

1

THE FACE OF DEATH

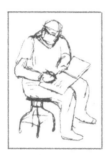

✢ ✢ ✢ ✢ ✢

CASE HISTORY: THE TUNNEL

Our hospital is divided into two buildings: one, antiquated but still in use, was constructed about 1900; the other, more modern, was built in the 1950s. Some integral parts of the hospital, for example, the Emergency Room (E.R.) and the morgue, are located in the old building, whereas other essential sections, including the Intensive Care Unit (I.C.U.) and the Coronary Care Unit (C.C.U), are in the new building. The buildings are linked by an underground tunnel.

Because of this haphazard arrangement, patients often have to be transported through the tunnel from the old building to the new one. That is, many patients brought in on an emergency basis—someone with a suspected heart attack, for instance—must be admitted through the E.R. in the old building and then conveyed on a stretcher to the new building via the tunnel.

This tunnel is like no other. It is long and narrow (approximately one and one-half city blocks from end to end and two stretchers wide). Its gray cement floor looks worn, as though scarred with the weight of all the feet and wheels that have hurried over its sunless surface. Yellowish rectangular tiles line the walls. Their jaundiced appearance recalls the pollution-tainted tiles of tunnels found beneath rivers, but here there are no cars or honking horns or smiling faces in vehicles, no policemen standing guard along the walls, no tollmen. No visible tollmen, at any rate. Yet, either before or after this tunnel, a toll is certainly taken.

The traffic through this subterranean passageway, as you have surmised correctly, is exceedingly strange. Though it is assuredly physical, a combination of bodies and equipment, it is also almost eerily ethereal. One might expect to see ghosts or phantoms curling through the corridor.

The ambience in this lower roadway—this *via inferna*, as the ancients might say—is heavy, congested, and oppressive. It is difficult to breathe even if you are healthy and not in distress like the patient on the stretcher. The only sound you hear is the droning of the ventilation fan. You wonder if it is really working, the air of this place is so stale. There are no windows, but it is bright. Fluorescent tubes fling down light from above and make you squint. Except for one curve, the tunnel is straight. If you stare directly ahead, you think you are caught in an almost endless tube.

The interns in our hospital hate this tunnel, curse it, dread it, and must travel through it time and time again. They loathe it for good reason. When an intern "on call" in the new building is assigned a new patient who is considered critically ill (e.g., someone being sent to the I.C.U. or C.C.U.), he must go through the tunnel, pick up his patient in the E.R., and accompany him, through the tunnel, to the new building. Thus, the intern has to make this terrible trip twice: once without his patient and once with him. Because the patient is probably gravely ill, he is hooked up to all sorts of life-sustaining and life-monitoring equipment, for example, a cardiac monitor and intravenous poles and perhaps some other emergency gear. There is also a defibrillator in case the patient has a cardiac arrest. The incessant nightmare of every intern in our hospital is that his patient's heart will stop or his patient will stop breathing in that tunnel, for the intern knows that when he is in there, he himself is the only medical person he can call on for help. In fact, an intern is so isolated in the tunnel that, even if he is perfectly healthy, he feels at times as though he is going to his own grave.

One Intern's Tale

It is around 2:00 A.M. I am on call in the new building. About an hour ago I managed to lie down on the bed in the on-call room. I closed my eyes, shuttered my ears, and tried to turn off my brain. Just as I am beginning to slide into the healing oblivion of sleep, I get a call. I have to pick up a patient in the E.R. He is having chest pains and must be admitted to the C.C.U. to rule out a myocardial infarction.

Gathering up my nerves and my tired brain, I descend into the tunnel not knowing whether this will be just another routine case or an "interesting" (i.e., unusual or complicated) one. You never know. The unexpected is always expectable in the hospital routine.

At times, an intern actually hopes for an interesting case: one from which he may learn something new or see something that a doctor does not see every day, if ever. But not at 2:00 A.M. When it is probably the intern's last admission for the night (the new intern starts admitting at 8:00 A.M.), he hopes that at this unholy hour any admission he has to take will be just a simple, routine one—a rule-out infarction, the chest pains turning out to be indigestion.

I hurry through the tunnel. As soon as I reach the E.R., I begin taking my patient's medical history. I have to get the basic facts and begin my evaluation. I must also arrange for support to transfer my patient to the new building, notify the C.C.U. about the admission, and give the nurses there a brief description of the case. All of this takes about twenty minutes.

What strikes me immediately about my new patient, Mr. B, age forty-five, is that he seems frightened to death. As I take his history, I realize that he has some good reason for his terror. First, although he has already been given some morphine, he is having what we doctors call a moderate amount of chest pain. (Never mind that a patient might call it a terrible, excruciating, or unbearable amount of pain, as might a doctor-patient experiencing it.) Second, his electrocardiogram is abnormal, and he knows it. Third, I learn that eight or ten months before, in Boston, Mr. B had had a very severe heart attack during which he had almost died. In sum, Mr. B knows what a bad heart attack is; he knows how close to death he had come. He therefore understands fully the gravity of his chest pain right now. And he is terrified.

One of the crucial functions of the intern during those first few minutes in the E.R. is to make his patient feel confident of three major things: (1) he is in good hands (even though those hands may be trembling), (2) his pain will be relieved, and (3) things will work out. All are particularly important for a heart attack patient. The intern certainly does not want him to worry or feel uncomfortable because anxiety and pain can aggravate his condition. The intern wants his heart attack patient to feel as relaxed as possible.

Mr. B and I are now ready to start through the tunnel. Although I have tried to reassure him and make him feel relaxed, he is still very tense. He appears petrified—almost literally. His face seems to say that this is the end for him, that he is sure he is dying here and now.

We start through the tunnel. Mr. B is hooked up to all sorts of life-monitoring gear. The cardiac monitor, another kind of telltale heart, keeps pounding the air with its nervous pulsations. There are only three of us in the tunnel: Mr. B and I, and the attendant pushing the stretcher.

About halfway through, appearing almost like an apparition, I can see coming toward us from the other end a strange configuration that I cannot clearly make out at first. I think I can discern a caravan of several black-clad shapes advancing very slowly. Mr. B does not see anything yet because he is lying flat on his stretcher. As they approach, the faraway figures become more distinct. I realize that the procession is composed of a number of bearded fellows garbed in black hats and black outfits—everything about them seems black. Behind the men and moving slowly, as if weighted down by some unbearable burden, is a stretcher completely covered in white. A few small bumps protrude from beneath its sheeted surface. All at once, I know this stretcher can be bearing but one thing: a corpse draped in a sheet. This realization is quite startling, even to me, because I know that the bodies of patients who die in our hospital are generally taken to the morgue, by stretcher, in the hospital's blue boxes. Am I hallucinating? The caravan seems to be unreal. Its mournful and foreboding mien makes it look like a cortege from hell. It is terrifying to me, and I am perfectly sound.

The first thing I think is that Mr. B will not see this procession. But when it reaches us, Mr. B's stretcher and the corpse-laden stretcher almost touch, and we have to slow down. The tunnel is just wide enough for the two stretchers to inch cautiously past each other. As we decelerate, Mr. B turns his head slightly to the left and sees passing alongside him—so close he could have touched it had he but extended his hand—the spectral stretcher with its white-cloaked corpse. It even seems to me, when the two stretchers are parallel, that they halt right next to each other. On the one side is my patient, whose body and face are frozen with fear; on the other side, facing and exactly parallel to Mr. B, is the sheet-covered corpse.

No one says a word. Only the cardiac monitor throbs into the silence. Time and breath seem to stand still. While all this is happening (does it last minutes or only seconds? it seems an eternity), I keep looking at Mr. B. He is still as stone. At last he looks up at me. And I know, from nothing but the expression on his face, that he believes he has just seen an image of himself.

We do not talk. We barely breathe.

After I have gotten Mr. B settled into the C.C.U., I do my write-up on him. I notice that I feel particularly exhausted.

It must be dawn.

About two days pass. Mr. B is doing well and resting comfortably. It turns out that he was indeed having another heart attack the night he was admitted. But he would survive it and leave the hospital.

I check on Mr. B several times a day. We have not spoken about what we saw in the tunnel. Suddenly, as I am about to leave his room after having just examined him, he says, "Doctor, remember that night you brought me in? That was a dead body, wasn't it?"

I cannot escape answering. "Yes, it was," I respond.

That is all that happened. We did not talk more about it, then or ever.

After a few weeks, Mr. B went home. But his face and that scene in the tunnel stayed with me after he left and are with me even now, years later. For I think that if ever a patient with a legitimate reason for fearing his own death actually came face to face with the embodiment of his fear, it happened then. I am sure that almost every patient in the hospital worries to some extent about his own death, but that worry is usually an abstraction, not a concrete, palpable figure. That night, however, just when Mr. B thought he was dying there on that hospital stretcher, he actually faced and all but touched the image of his own death. His pain-carved, petrified face could have marked, during those moments shrouded in an unspeakable silence, his own tombstone.

Sometime later I learned more about the mysterious procession we had seen. The black parade—the kind of ghostly convoy you might conjure up in a nightmare—was actually a group of religious Jews accompanying an orthodox rabbi who had died. I sought out a rabbi and asked him if he could explain the meaning of such a ritual caravan.

The rabbi said that the deceased must have been a revered *rebbe*, a Hasidic rabbi, to have merited such special attention. The men were accompanying his body as a mark of esteem for a scholar of the Torah. When they kept vigil over his body or walked with it, they were probably reciting prayer softly or silently, such as these words from Genesis 3:19 and the Twenty-third Psalm: "for dust thou art, and unto dust shalt thou return"; "Yea, though I walk through the valley of the shadow of death, I will fear no evil: for thou art with me." According to the rabbi, the corpse probably was draped in a sheet, instead of encased in one of the hospital's blue boxes, because the men wished to follow in some way their shtetl's burial custom. He added that he had never witnessed such a procession. Neither had I, of course; nor have I seen anything like it since. In fact, since that night I have not seen any sort of procession passing through that tunnel. But the memory of the cortege and my patient's face continues to haunt me every time I walk through it.

✝ ✝ ✝ ✝ ✝

LITERARY PARALLELS

How have some other people confronted the face of death? We do not have to go far to find what we seek; some of the finest, fullest, and richest depictions of such encounters are found in literature. From time immemorial, man has questioned, contemplated, and sought to come to terms with his own mortality. "Wonders are many on earth, and the greatest of these / Is man. . . . / For every ill he hath found its remedy / Save only death," wrote Sophocles.[1] To try to see death through another person's eyes is particularly appropriate—and particularly painful—in our death-denying society. But our running away, as Shakespeare so wittily said, makes us but "death's fool": "Merely, thou art death's fool; / For him thou labour'st by thy flight to shun, / And yet runn'st toward him still."[2]

MONTAIGNE AND THE
DIALOGUE BETWEEN DEATH AND LIFE

French philosopher and essayist Michel de Montaigne (1533–1592) did not flee from the face of death. In fact, his earliest essays frequently sound the theme of man's mortality. "To philosophize is to learn to die," he wrote sometime between 1572 and 1574. "The goal of our career is death. It is the necessary object of our aim. . . . Let us have nothing on our minds as often as death. . . . Premeditation of death is premeditation of freedom."[3]

Several events help to account for Montaigne's early preoccupation with death. The years from 1563 to 1573 were marred for him by the deaths of numerous people who were close to him, including his father, his closest friend, an uncle, a brother, and two infant daughters. These years were also marked by the deaths of thousands of Frenchmen killed in the religious civil wars that were to wrack France for the rest of the century. He wrote, "With such frequent and ordinary examples passing before our eyes, how can we pos-

sibly rid ourselves of the thought of death and of the idea
that at every moment it is gripping us by the throat?"[4]

Perhaps it is ironic, but chronic illness helped wean
Montaigne from his fear of, and preoccupation with, death.
In the summer of 1578, when he was forty-five, he was first
afflicted with bladder and kidney stones. "I am at grips with
the worst of all maladies, the most sudden, the most painful,
the most mortal, and the most irremediable," he lamented
in his essay "Of the Resemblance of Children to Fathers."[5]
His father, whom he had adored, had been "extraordinarily
afflicted" with the same disease and had died some sixteen
years before.[6] Nevertheless, even in his affliction, Montaigne
managed to find some consolation. "I have at least this profit
from the stone, that it will complete what I have still not
been able to accomplish in myself and reconcile and
familiarize me completely with death: for the more my illness oppresses and bothers me, the less will death be something for me to fear," he wrote in the same essay, around
1579–80.[7]

At just about this time—about a year after the onset of
his illness—Montaigne completely changed his ideas about
philosophy. No longer would he say, as he had just a few
years before, that "to philosophize is to learn to die." Now he
would proclaim "it is philosophy that teaches us to live."[8]

In 1580, Montaigne set out for seventeen months of travel
to the sights and mineral baths of Germany, Switzerland,
and Italy (where he had an audience with Pope Gregory
III). His travels, as well as his experiences with his persistent
illness, helped shape his philosophy. His new outlook on
death—and life—is evident in the entry in his *Travel Journal* dated 24 August 1581. He was then at La Villa, a mineral
bath near Lucca, Italy, recovering from one of his worst
attacks of renal colic. "There would be too much weakness
and cowardice on my part if, finding myself every day in a
position to die in this manner, I did not make every effort
toward being able to bear death lightly as soon as it sur-

prised me. And in the meantime it will be wise to accept joyously the good that it pleases God to send us."[9]

Advancing age, too, made Montaigne value life more dearly. In his final essay, "Of Experience," composed about four years before he died, he wrote, "I enjoy . . . [life] twice as much as others, for the measure of enjoyment depends on the greater or lesser attention that we lend it. Especially at this moment, when I perceive that mine is so brief in time, I try to increase it in weight; I try to arrest the speed of its flight by the speed with which I grasp it. The shorter my possession of life, the deeper and fuller I must make it."[10]

In the dialogue between death and life, therefore, the richly human voice of life triumphed at the time of Montaigne's death: facing death had taught him to love living. "If we have known how to live steadfastly and tranquilly, we shall know how to die in the same way," he wrote during his last years.[11] Montaigne's wisdom holds true for modern times.

But what if a person has not known how to live steadfastly or tranquilly? And what if when that person becomes fatally ill, he cannot face his fear of dying or even the fact that he is dying? Such is the case of Ivan Ilych.

"THE DEATH OF IVAN ILYCH"

In Tolstoy's ground-breaking story published in 1886, we can see the lessons of Montaigne as well as some of the insights of modern psychiatry as described by Elisabeth Kübler-Ross (in *On Death and Dying*) and others. For what the reader experiences in "The Death of Ivan Ilych" is the anguish of a dying patient who has not been able to express—to verbalize and thus to cast out—his fear of death. And because he has not been able to express his anguish, Ivan Ilych's dying is a torture for everyone around him and, most of all, for himself.

"Ivan Ilych's life had been most simple and most ordinary and therefore most terrible," Tolstoy says in introducing him.[12] He had been a judge and had died at the age of forty-five. All his life Ivan Ilych had pursued "successes"—financial, social, and professional—and to a certain degree he had achieved all three. Yet something was seriously wrong. For one thing, his marriage was a shambles. His wife had come to hate him and even to wish him dead, but "she did not want him to die because then his salary would cease. And this irritated her against him still more."[13]

Then Ivan Ilych had become ill. There was a pain in his left side, a terrible taste in his mouth. Finally, he had consulted a doctor. What Ivan Ilych most wanted to know was, "was his case serious or not? But the doctor ignored that inappropriate question. From the doctor's point of view, the real question was to decide between a floating kidney, chronic catarrh, or appendicitis."[14] As he paid the physician, Ivan Ilych ventured rather timidly, "But tell me, in general, is this complaint dangerous or not?"[15] The doctor did not deign to answer; instead, he looked at Ivan Ilych "sternly ... with one eye," in just the same way that Ivan Ilych the judge had so often looked at recalcitrant prisoners in his courtroom.

As Ivan Ilych's condition worsened, other doctors were consulted. But no one, including the doctors, would admit to him that he was dying. One time, however, Ivan Ilych overheard his wife talking to a friend. And all at once he began to realize the truth.

> "No, you are exaggerating!" [his wife] ... was saying.
>
> "Exaggerating! Don't you see it? Why, he's a dead man! Look at his eyes—there's no light in them. But what is it that is wrong with him?"
>
> "No one knows...."
>
> Suddenly ... [Ivan Ilych's] heart sank and he felt dazed. "My God! my God!" he muttered.... And suddenly the matter presented itself in a quite different aspect.... "It's not a ques-

tion of appendix or kidney, but of life and ... death." ... A chill came over him, his breathing ceased, and he felt only the throbbing of his heart.[16]

From then on, Ivan Ilych was in continual despair. At first, he tried to deny that he was dying. "Not only was he not accustomed to the thought, he simply did not and could not grasp it."[17]

He sought to combat his terror by going to work. But more and more, he was forced to face "*It*": that which he could not, would not, and dared not name.

> He would say to himself: "I will take up my duties again. . . ." And banishing all doubts he would go to the law courts. . . . But suddenly in the midst of those proceedings the pain in his side ... would begin its own gnawing work. Ivan Ilych would turn his attention to it and try to drive the thought of it away, but without success. *It* would come and stand before him and look at him, and he would be petrified and the light would die out of his eyes, and he would again begin asking himself whether *It* alone was true. And ... [he would] return home with the sorrowful consciousness that his judicial labors could not as formerly hide from him what he wanted them to hide, and could not deliver him from *It*. And what was worst of all was that *It* drew his attention to itself not in order to make him take some action but only that he should look at *It*, look it straight in the face: look at it and without doing anything, suffer inexpressibly.
>
> And to save himself from this condition Ivan Ilych looked for consolations—new screens— ... but then they immediately fell to pieces or rather became transparent, as if *It* penetrated them and nothing could veil *It*. . . . [Finally, Ivan Ilych] would go to his study, lie down, and again be alone with *It*: face to face with *It*. And nothing could be done with *It* except to look at it and shudder.[18]

For months, Ivan Ilych faced the face of death in this way, and during all that time everyone around him tried to pretend that he was only ill, not dying. He, too, participated in that deception, though it tortured him. "What tormented Ivan Ilych most was the deception . . .—their not wishing to admit what they all knew and what he knew, but wanting to lie to him concerning his terrible condition, and wishing and forcing him to participate in that lie."[19]

Left alone with his doubts and fears, Ivan Ilych, the former judge, began to judge not only the people around him but also himself. The "falsity around him and within him did more than anything else to poison his last days."[20] Still, Ivan Ilych could not condemn his past or himself. "'Maybe I did not live as I ought to have done,' it suddenly occurred to him. 'But how could that be, when I did everything properly?' he replied, and immediately dismissed from his mind this, the sole solution of all the riddles of life and death, as something quite impossible."[21]

His sufferings increased.

> Ivan Ilych's physical sufferings were terrible, but worse than the physical sufferings were his mental sufferings, which were his chief torture.

> His mental sufferings were due to the fact that that night, as he looked at . . . [his peasant servant's] sleepy, good-natured face . . . , the question suddenly occurred to him: "What if my whole life has really been wrong?" . . .

> In the morning when he saw first his footman, then his wife, then his daughter, and then a doctor, their every word and movement confirmed to him the awful truth that had been revealed to him during the night. In them he saw himself— all that for which he had lived—and saw clearly that it was not real at all, but a terrible and huge deception which had hidden both life and death.[22]

Ivan Ilych spent his last three days screaming. The noise was "so terrible that one could not hear it through two closed doors without horror."[23] It had begun quite suddenly. His wife sent for the priest, and Ivan Ilych took communion.

His wife came in to congratulate him after his communion, and when uttering the usual conventional words she added:

"You feel better, don't you?"

Without looking at her he said "Yes."

Her dress, her figure, the expression of her face, the tone of her voice, all revealed the same thing. "This is wrong, it is not as it should be. All you have lived for and still live for is falsehood and deception, hiding life and death from you." And as soon as he admitted that thought, his hatred and his agonizing physical suffering again sprang up, and with that suffering a consciousness of the unavoidable, approaching end. . . .

"Go away! Go away and leave me alone!" [he shouted].

From that moment the screaming began that continued for three days. . . . At the moment he answered his wife he realized that he was lost, that there was no return, that the end had come, the very end, and his doubts were still unsolved and remained doubts.[24]

On the third day, however, Ivan Ilych opened his eyes to find his young son kissing his hand. In that moment Ivan Ilych suddenly felt sorry for others, even for his wife. And in that instant he was freed from his fear of death.

He sought his former accustomed fear of death and did not find it. "Where is it? What death?" There was no fear because there was no death.

In place of death there was light.

"So that's what it is?" he suddenly exclaimed aloud. "What joy!"[25]

His burst of love, which is human and/or divine, had freed him from his fear and had freed him to face—and embrace—his death with a feeling of "joy."

Two hours later he died.

Something rattled in his throat, his emaciated body twitched,
then the gasping and rattle became less and less frequent.
"It is finished!" said someone near him.
He heard these words and repeated them in his soul.
"Death is finished," he said to himself. "It is no more!"
He drew in a breath, stopped in the midst of a sigh, stretched
out, and died.[26]

Whether one interprets these final words of the story in a
secular or a religious light, it is clear that for Ivan Ilych and
for Tolstoy death loses its terror when the person who is
dying is able to care and feel for others instead of just for
himself. The face of death no longer appears fearful in the
face of love—divine or human—because, in loving, the
dying person believes that he is part of something greater
than himself.

Is love the answer then? Can love always conquer the
fear of death? We decided to examine how feelings of erotic
and/or spiritual love are expressed in some twentieth-century depictions of facing death in war.

LOVE, SEX, AND DEATH

William Butler Yeats wrote "An Irish Airman Foresees His
Death" in 1918. The speaker in the poem is Major Robert
Gregory, a thirty-seven-year-old Irish painter, scholar, and
horseman who fought with the English in the Royal Flying
Corps; he was killed in action on the Italian front on January
13, 1918.

In Yeats's poem, indifference—or rather, apparent indifference that actually masks a deep anger about the futility
of life—characterizes the airman's attitude toward death.
His emotions are numbed, the airman reveals, because he
fights neither for "love" of the English nor for "hate" of the
enemy. In addition, he believes that nothing he can do either
in living or in dying can help those he really wants to help:
his poor, oppressed Irish countrymen.

> I know that I shall meet my fate
> Somewhere among the clouds above;
> Those that I fight I do not hate,
> Those that I guard I do not love;
> My country is Kiltartan Cross,
> My countrymen Kiltartan's poor,
> No likely end could bring them loss,
> Or leave them happier than before.

Still, the airman says, something drives him on; some almost erotic "impulse of delight" propels him to seek out death in the skies. What urges him on in his "lonely" questing for great pleasure or great joy is, perhaps, his drive to overcome his feelingless state and his depression. Yet he does not deceive himself about what he can accomplish because everything, he says, appears to him a "waste": his past, his future, were he to continue living, and his death.

> Nor law, nor duty bade me fight,
> Nor public men, nor cheering crowds,
> A lonely impulse of delight
> Drove to this tumult in the clouds;
> I balanced all, brought all to mind,
> The years to come seemed waste of breath,
> A waste of breath the years behind
> In balance with this life, this death.[27]

His death is a waste because his life seems to him to be a waste. And his quasi-erotic embracing of death is not an expression of love; it is a manifestation of his anger at, and despair in, life.

Sometimes facing death in war is portrayed as a heroic and truly loving experience. Such is Katow's death in André Malraux's *The Human Condition* (*La Condition humaine,* often translated as *Man's Fate*).

The scene is China, 1927. Katow, a Russian, has been fighting with the Communists. A seasoned revolutionary who had served five years of hard labor in Russia, fought in the Russian Revolution of 1917, and had even been shot by a firing squad, Katow is now a prisoner with many others. All are condemned to die. Some are to be shot. Important participants in the insurrection, including Katow and his friend Kyo, are to be burned alive in the boiler of a locomotive. A whistle blows. Each time it sounds, another prisoner has been burned to death.

Wounded, lying on the floor in the dark, Katow feels his friend Kyo dead beside him. Kyo has just swallowed his cyanide tablet; in that way he has escaped death in the locomotive. Near him Katow hears two young Chinese revolutionaries crying. Suddenly, he makes the most difficult decision of his life: he will give them his cyanide. It is not that he does not suffer, nor is it that he does not fear the fiery death that awaits him. In fact, he feels terribly alone and frightened. "But a man could be stronger than that solitude and even, perhaps, than that atrocious whistle; fear fought within him against the most terrible temptation of his life."[28] Then he breaks his cyanide in half and gives the pieces to the two terrified boys. It is a "gift of more than his life."[29]

There is a terrifying, sickening moment when the pieces of cyanide are lost as one boy tries to pass the poison to the other. During the frantic, surreptitious searching, one boy's hand grasps Katow's and clings to it. "Katow, also, squeezed that hand; he was on the verge of tears, caught up in this pitiable faceless fraternity . . . given to him in this darkness in exchange for the greatest gift he had ever given, and which was given perhaps in vain. Although Souen [one of the boys] continued to search, the two hands remained joined." Finally, the pieces are found. Katow "gave them back,—squeezed even harder that hand which sought once more for his hand, and he waited, his shoulders trembling, his teeth clacking. . . . The hand he was holding suddenly twisted his hand. . . . He envied that convulsive suffocation." After the boys have died, Katow lies on his stomach and waits. "The trembling of his shoulders did not cease."[30]

When he is marched outside by the soldiers, Katow tries

to bolster his courage. "Come on! let's pretend that I died in a fire," he tells himself. He is shoved toward, and into, the boiler. "All [the prisoners'] heads . . . followed the rhythm of his walk, with love, with terror, with resignation."[31] For at least two reasons, Katow's fear-filled yet fearless confrontation with death assumes heroic proportions: he believes in the cause for which he has lived and for which he is dying, and he is able to give of himself to others in a supremely selfless act. He discovers, in squeezing that grateful, fearful hand offered to him in the darkness, a feeling of fraternity that is at once sensuous and spiritual.

Often, however, death in war is depicted not as a love act but as a perversion of love, an obscenity. Such is the case in *Obscenities,* Michael Casey's book about the Vietnam War which won the Yale Series of Younger Poets' Award in 1972. "On Death" transmits that revulsion:

> School children walk by
> Some stare
> Some keep on walking
> Some adults stare too
> With handkerchiefs
> Over their nose
> A woman
> Sits on the pavement
> Beside
> Waits
> And pounds her fists
> On pavement
> Flies all over
> It   like made of wax
> No jaw
> Intestines poured
> Out of the stomach
> The penis in the air
>   It won't matter then to me   but now
> I don't want in death to be a
> Public obscenity like this[32]

In these three cases, where facing death in war aroused some kind of love feelings or a perversion thereof, the face of death for each fighter resembled the face of life as he saw it: bitter indifference for the airman; a worthy, selfless cause for Katow; and a lewd, repulsive horror for Casey ("If you have a farm in Vietnam / And a house in hell / Sell the farm / And go home."[33]) Love combats the fear of death, then, only if one can feel love. But in war, which is an extreme situation (just as facing death at any time is an extreme situation), the feelings of love may, or may not, come or help. After all, even Katow, whose love feelings were far more exalted than the airman's or Casey's, felt fear.

In war there is the implication that facing death means facing a violent or sudden death. But facing a less rapid death—for example, facing death from a slow-killing disease—may evoke some very different reactions that may also call forth, in their own ways, some equally haunting visions of love. Following are the cases of two people who know they will die of cancer, probably within one year.

CANCER WARD AND "A SPLENDID DAY"

Dontsova is a doctor in Solzhenitsyn's *Cancer Ward*. "For thirty years she had been dealing with other people's illnesses, and for a good twenty she had sat in front of the X-ray screen. She had read the screen, read the film, read the distorted, imploring eyes of her patients."[34] And now she has become a patient.

> The moment she admitted the disease existed, she was crushed by it like a frog under foot. Adjusting to the disease was at first unbearable. Her world had capsized. . . . She was not yet dead, and yet she had to give up her husband, her son, her daughter, her grandson, and her medical work as well, even though it was her own work, medicine, that would be rolling over her and through her like a noisy train.[35]

During her X-ray examination by other doctors, Dontsova refuses to look at the most important X-ray. She feels frightened and depleted. Her worst fears are confirmed: she has cancer of the esophagus. Immediately, her perspective of life changes. "It had once occurred to her that there was a lack of color, joy, festivity in her life—it was all work and worry, work and worry. But how wonderful the old life seemed now! Parting with it was so unthinkable it made her scream."[36]

Before she is sent to another clinic for treatment, Dontsova continues to work. But she is constantly plagued by the thought that in "a few days' time she would be lying in a hospital bed, as helpless and dumb as . . . [her own patients] were, neglecting her appearance, awaiting the pronouncements of her more experienced seniors, afraid of the pain."[37] And as she talks with a patient, she wonders "whether or not he would live out the year. In fact, he and she were in the same position."[38]

Powerfully, Solzhenitsyn makes the reader feel Dontsova's fears about her disease and her dying. Just as grippingly, he makes us experience her refound love of life— the very life she had once considered so colorless and tedious.

"A Splendid Day," an essay by Molly Ingle Michie, a forty-six-year-old housewife, offers another view of a person facing death from cancer. Between the diagnosis of her lung cancer ("broncho-alveolar cell carcinoma")[39] and her death, Michie lived nine months. What is remarkable about the essay, what makes it virtually unique in the thousands of pages of literature devoted to death and dying, is her humor, which she constantly juxtaposes with powerful, often sentimental, emotions. Indeed, it is Michie's mingling of the humorous with the serious and sentimental which gives her perspective on dying so much distance, depth, and richness.

Michie begins almost coldly, objectively. "The surgeon did not pussyfoot around about the likelihood of my dying. He said that half the people with my disease were alive one year after diagnosis. Only three out of a hundred were alive five years later."[40] And so, she writes, diverting herself—and us—from her pain, that night "I scribbled down a list of dreaded tasks that I would never have to do again—(1) give large dinner parties, (2) clean the oven, (3) scrub floors, (4) wash delicate things by hand, (5) remove stains." Already her humor has distanced her, and us, from her dying. In so doing it enables us to come closer to her without our own anxieties about death hindering our relationship.

Drawing up a list of "things to be glad about while dying of cancer," Michie interlaces humor with nostalgia: "(1) I don't have to worry about getting cancer anymore. (2) I had a wonderful trip to Jamaica. (3) I don't have to worry about gray hair. I don't have to worry about rosacea." In the same vein, she found "two *real* benefits. (1) I found out that people love me who I would never have guessed loved me. I would have died without knowing. (2) I won't have to learn the metric system."[41]

Humor intertwines with anger in Michie's description of how she first coped with the knowledge that she would need radiation therapy for her cancer. As a young woman, she had developed "a full-blown, somewhat irrational phobia about X-rays."[42] And now, she herself would have to be "sizzled" with thousands of rads. She knew her anger about dying needed to be expressed. That anger, she found,

> came in a strange free floating form. There *must* be someone to blame, someone who robbed me of precious time—the very prime of my life. My anger, free floating, gradually took an animal form. A tiny albino falcon appeared over the door of my hospital room, a vicious fellow with pink eyes and long pink talons. I named him A.F., which stood for Albino Falcon and for Anger, Free Floating. He was ready to attack anyone who abused me in any way—callous nurses, bearers of inedible meals, inconsiderate visitors, or cleaning personnel who might wake me from a nap.... For four days no one was callous or careless. A.F. was getting frantic and larger. He began flapping wildly around the room. Clearly he would have to attack an innocent, if a proper villain could not be found soon.[43]

But then Michie was told that she needed radiation treatments. "A.F. and I were jubilant—a perfect villain! A.F. and I settled down, he to sharpen his talons and I to ponder my hatred of radiation and all doctors and technicians who practiced it."[44] But all Michie's fears and angers about radiation are counterbalanced by her final statement regarding it. The "radiotherapy department ... was ... full of talented, dedicated people who had given me months full of happy hours, months that I could not have expected from any other course of treatment."[45]

Because of Michie's own attitudes and actions, and because, as she said, her family and friends were supportive—"letting me talk and helping me put my thoughts and things in order"—she found in her slow and relatively painless dying "an enormous satisfaction—a summing up."[46] Her humorous summing up of the things she did not like in life and her nostalgic summing up of the things she did love (including family, friends, beauty, and life itself) made facing death less fearful and more fulfilling for her than for most people. By using humor to diffuse her anger and to distance herself from life—and so from death—Michie was able to provide a nostalgic and grateful portrait of a life worth living and of a death lived fully in the dying.

A SUMMING UP

As we reflect on Mr. B, the patient in the case history, and the literary selections, we are forced to face that from which we—both physicians and laymen—generally wish to flee: death. Yet, we realize, since no matter what we do in life each of us will eventually have to face the prospect of his or her own death—although probably not so dramatically as Mr. B. did the night he encountered in the constricted tunnel that sheet-draped corpse with its black cortege—we ought at least to think about death from time to time, with-

out, however, becoming obsessed by it. As we have shown,
there are numerous, probably innumerable, ways of facing
death. But one thing was present in each of these cases of
a person facing death—the vision of life, death's opposite.
It is that which we must learn to appreciate and savor before
the clock runs out.

> Clock! sinister, frightful, impassive god, whose finger
> Shakes at us and says to us: *"Remember!*
> Vibrant Pains in your fear-filled heart
> Will soon plant themselves as in a target;
>
> Vaporous Pleasure towards the horizon will flee
> Like a sylphid into the theater's wing; voraciously
> Each instant eats from you a morsel of the delight given
> To each man for the duration of his season.
>
> Three thousand six hundred times
> An hour, the Second whispers: *Remember!*—Fast,
> With her insect's voice, Now says: I am the Past,
> And with my foul proboscis I've sucked up your life!
>
> *Souviens-toi! Remember!* prodigal, *Esto
> Memor!* (My metal throat speaks all languages.)
> The minutes, frolicsome mortal, are gangues
> You must not leave without extracting their gold!
>
> *Remember* that Time is a greedy gambler who wins
> Without cheating, at each turn! that's the rule. Day is waning;
> Night is rising; *remember!* the abyss
> Is always thirsty; the water clock is draining.
>
> Soon the hour will strike when Chance divine,
> When august Virtue, your still virgin wife,
> When even Repentance (oh! the last inn!) will say
> To you: Die, old coward! It is too late!"[47]

2

MY CADAVER

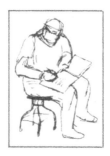

✛ ✛ ✛ ✛ ✛

CASE HISTORY

I had never intended to become a doctor. Because I had majored
in physics in college and then had earned a Ph.D. in nuclear physics, I had fulfilled only the bare minimum requirements in biology,
a one-year college course, when I entered medical school. Until
anatomy class began, therefore, all my previous experience with
dissecting animals had consisted of one frog.

The course in anatomy was a cultural shock for me, to say the
least. Most memorable was that our medical school actually scheduled a time for students to meet their cadavers. This was before
anatomy class actually began so that students could become fa-
miliarized with the place.

I remember going up alone, clutching the little card with my
cadaver's table number. Just walking into that room was surreal-
istic. I was greeted by row after row of dead bodies—about twenty-
five in all. They were covered up, of course, but it didn't make
any difference. I knew *what* they were. As I stood alone in that
room, I almost expected all those cadavers to get up and start

running after me. I found my cadaver at last, then quickly left. I didn't want to stay around.

During the first few weeks of formal anatomy classes, my classmates and I were relatively subdued and a bit tense, for obvious reasons: respect for the dead, a feeling of awe for this historical drama of dissection which only a privileged few had been sanctioned to perform, and so forth. We worked in groups: four students to a single cadaver. Each group remained with its cadaver for the whole course. Although you never knew who your cadaver was (you could find out your cadaver's name, but I never did), as the year went by, you tended to speculate about what kind of person your cadaver had been. You would look for clues in the anatomy—facial expression, general stature, hands, age, weight.

During our months of anatomy class, all of us probably developed intimate fantasies about our cadavers. This may seem peculiar, but I suppose we did it to give our cadavers life. I decided that my cadaver had been a kindly old woman who had read the classics, knew very little about science, and had been a widow for about twenty years. I also had the feeling that she had worked, perhaps editing books. Because she had scoliosis, I inferred that she had suffered from back pain, often took aspirin, and was probably not athletic. I did not think that she had had any children. I even imagined her walking down the street. In fact, sometimes when I was out walking, I would see someone who reminded me of my cadaver—a woman of seventy or so, a little bent over—and I would feel as though I knew her well.

As the year progressed, we became more relaxed in class. Dissecting the cadaver became more of a commonplace, just something we did every day, a job. Like so many things in medicine, the bizarre and extraordinary become ordinary and routine. For example, having just finished chopping up a lung, we would barely remember to wash our hands before going out to lunch. Naturally, every time you ate your lunch, your hands so reeked of formaldehyde that after a while you went around smelling like your cadaver. In a strange way, then, your cadaver and you became almost one.

Carrying this experience to the logical extreme (how can you judge if something is logical or illogical when you have spent months dissecting another human being's body?), the last day of anatomy class was traditionally a day of celebration. This was a complete contrast to the first day, when we had all been rather timid, respectful, and awed. Some of my fellow medical students brought in wine and champagne, and most of us spent the time laughing and drinking. It was a kind of carousing among the corpses. The group next to mine used the open abdominal cavity of their cadaver as the bottle holder for their champagne.

+ + + + +

LITERARY PARALLELS

Because it seemed more than a little disturbing that so many future physicians had behaved in such a gross, grotesque manner in anatomy class, we wondered how some other people had acted when contemplating—let alone dissecting—a corpse. We sought insights from the past and the present.

THE CORPSE AT THE BANQUET

The ancient Egyptians, according to Herodotus, purposely contemplated the image of a corpse to spur themselves on to renewed sensuous and sensual enjoyment. "In social meetings among the rich, when the banquet is ended, a servant carries round to the several guests a coffin, in which there is a wooden image of a corpse, carved and painted to resemble nature as nearly as possible.... As he shows it to each guest in turn, the servant says, 'Gaze here, and drink and be merry; for when you die, such will you be.'"[1] The grotesqueness of such a display at a banquet was surpassed only by the reaction it was meant to solicit in the beholders: in the face of death, the heady and deliberate pursuit of pleasure.

MEMENTO MORI, *DANSE MACABRE,* AND CHARNEL HOUSES

The corpse was also an important symbol for Christians of the late Middle Ages. But unlike the ancient Egyptians, who were advised to pursue pleasure after contemplating a corpse, Christians of the fourteenth and fifteenth centuries were admonished by the death-depicting art and literature of their era to fear death and damnation and to think about their eternal salvation. "Memento mori," they were constantly warned, "Remember that you must die." A glance at what life was like during the times of François Villon (1432?–1463?), one of the finest poets of fifteenth-century France, may help explain this preoccupation with death and cadavers.

When Villon was born in Paris in 1431 or 1432, France had been besieged for about a century by famines, massacres, and the Hundred Years' War (Joan of Arc was burned in 1431). The country had been assaulted as well by plague, smallpox, and other illnesses, which continued to take their toll. In August 1438, Marie de France, daughter of Charles VI, died from the epidemic (probably of smallpox) that was beginning in spread to Paris. "All the doctors who made the post-mortem died too. . . . In the rest of the city more than 45,000 succumbed."[2]

During Villon's era, therefore, men were accustomed to contemplating death almost daily. Proximity did not make it less fearsome. Indeed, the art and literature of the day deliberately emphasized the terrifying aspects of death. From the end of the fourteenth century until well into the sixteenth century, tombs were "decorated with hideous images of naked, rotted corpses, their feet and fists rigid, their mouths gaping, their entrails devoured by worms."[3] When Cardinal Lagrange died in Avignon in 1402, his tomb (now displayed in the Musée Calvet, Avignon) bore a bas-relief of a mummified body—half skeleton and half decomposed corpse— and an inscription that warned, "Wretch, what reason hast thou to be proud? Ashes thou art, and soon thou wilt be like me, a fetid corpse, feeding ground for worms."[4] In this atmosphere of death and decay, the art and verses of the *danse macabre* flourished.

The medieval danse macabre—the dance of the dead or the dance of death—was an allegorical representation of death taking hold of people of all ranks and conditions. A cadaverlike figure of death was paired with each living person. The dead led the dance and were the only ones

depicted as dancing, while the living appeared almost lifeless, as though frozen in their tracks by fear. The purpose
of the dance was to edify through pictures and words: to
serve, in effect, as a memento mori.

In the fifteenth century, murals were a common form of
the danse macabre. In fact, "the most popular representation known to the Middle Ages" was the danse macabre
painted in 1424–25 on the inside wall of the cemetery of
the Holy Innocents (Les Saints-Innocents) in Paris.[5] This mural consisted of a long line of about thirty pictures depicting
the whole range of human society. In the verses accompanying the scenes, Death addressed each living person, and
each responded in turn. The voice of Death was didactic,
satiric, or ironic; for example, to the portly abbot, Death
said, "The fattest rot soonest."[6] Because the verses of this
danse macabre were very popular, they were translated into
"English, Low German, Latin . . . and Catalan."[7]

The Paris cemetery where this celebrated mural was
painted reveals much about fifteenth-century attitudes toward cadavers, for just above the famous danse macabre
were the charnel houses (or charnels), ossuaries of exhumed
human bones displayed for public view. As in many other
churchyards of the time, the charnels were built along the
cemetery's inside walls. After the fourteenth century and its
epidemic of the Black Death, the burial ground had become
overcrowded, and so the "custom . . . [had arisen] of dis-
interring the dead and putting their remains in charnel
houses to make room for newcomers. . . . [R]ich and poor
were treated alike."[8] Every day crowds of people saw the
disinterred bones in the charnels of the Holy Innocents because in the fifteenth century this cemetery, "the biggest and
best known in Paris,"[9] was not only a sacred burying ground
but also a forum, a public square, a marketplace, and a
promenade for prostitutes. "There were small booths below
the famous charnel houses, in which books, cloth, and iron-
mongery were sold. The vendors exposed their wares to the
public view on the tombs."[10] "You would find little shops
there near the charnel houses and prostitutes beneath the

arcades. . . . Even celebrations were held in that place. To such an extent had the horrible become familiar."[11]

Villon gives further insights into this cadaver-haunted era.

FRANÇOIS VILLON AND THE
"BALLADE OF THE HANGED MEN"

That Villon's poetry is haunted by figures of death is not surprising considering his era and his life. Although he had received bachelor's and master's degrees from the Faculty of Arts of the University of Paris (the latter making him a junior member of the clergy), the poet became a derelict, a thief, and the killer of a priest. After several imprisonments he was condemned at about age thirty to be "hanged and strangled" (*"pendu et estranglé"*).[12] He was reprieved, however, and banished from Paris for ten years. We have no record of what became of him after that.

In his poetry, Villon reveals his fears not only of death's physical aspects (e.g., how it destroys the human body) but also of hell. Here is how he depicts death's fearful physical effects on a cadaver:

> Death makes him shudder, turn pallid hues,
> Makes his veins grow taut and his nose sag,
> Makes his neck puff out and his skin flag;
> It lengthens and swells his joints and sinews.[13]

Elsewhere, however, the poet makes us see and feel his faith that if he repents, God will forgive and welcome him.

In some of his finest work, Villon actually makes us feel both his fear and his faith by means of shifting tones: now clinical, grotesque, or desensitized; now pathetic, imploring, or prayerful; now ironically humorous; now poignantly serious. In this way he evokes contradictory reactions in the reader: distance and closeness, coldness and compassion, a feeling of difference and a feeling of fraternity. Through his shifting tones, Villon at times makes his reader feel almost one with him. He does this, for example, in his famous "Ballade of the Hanged Men," often called "The Villon Epitaph."

Condemned to be hanged, the poet depicts himself and those hanged with him as cadavers decaying on the gibbet. The voice speaking throughout the ballade is that of the hanged men's cadavers.

BALLADE OF THE HANGED MEN

Human brothers who live when our lives are through,
Do not harden your hearts against us, for
If you have pity on us creatures poor,
The sooner will God have mercy on you.
You see us hanging here, five, six or so,
As for our flesh, which we nourished overmuch,
It grew rotten and was devoured long ago,
And we, the bones, are becoming ashes and dust.
Let no one laugh at our sad fall:
But pray that God absolve us all!

If we call you brothers, you should not be
Contemptuous, even though
We were killed by law. However, you know,
Not all men judge soberly;
Because we are dead, make our apology
To the son of the Virgin Mary,
So that He not staunch His grace for us,
Preserving us from hellfire fulminous.
We are dead; let no one catcall;
But pray that God absolve us all!

We've been drenched by the rain that purifies,
And by the sun blackened and desiccated:
Magpies and crows have gouged out our eyes
And our beards and eyebrows eradicated.
We're never seated at any time at all,
Transported now here, now there, unceasingly,
According to the wind's wanton call,
More pecked by birds than a thimble by a needle.
And so, do not join our confraternity;
But pray that God absolve us all!

Prince Jesus, who over us all has mastery,
Keep Hell from having our seigniory:

Let's have no debts or doings therewithal.
This, men, is not a jest at all;
But pray that God absolve us all![14]

While contemplating the image of his own cadaver, Villon mingles emotional distance with pathos, a clinical de-
tachment with a fraternal embracing of all men. Although
he believes that he will be hanged, he knows—and makes
his readers remember—that we shall all die (though not
necessarily on a gibbet), that our bodies will also grow rotten, and our bones become "ashes and dust." The "Ballade
of the Hanged Men" is, therefore, the poet-cadaver's lesson
to the living: we should see in the cadaver's state the image
of our own sorry—and inevitable—fate.

With the image of Villon's cadaver in mind, we thought
back to that anatomy class. And we began to wonder how
some physician-writers had reacted to contact with, or contemplation of, the cadaver.

FRANÇOIS RABELAIS

François Rabelais (1494?–1553) was a Doctor of Medicine
and practicing physician, an ordained priest, the father of
three illegitimate children, and the author of the famed
comic saga *Gargantua and Pantagruel.* He received his medical doctorate from, and for a time taught at, the Montpellier
Faculty of Medicine, which was, along with the Paris Faculty
of Medicine, the best in France at that time.

During Rabelais's era, the church was very powerful
and, in general, against innovation. The "Sorbonne—the
dominant Faculty of Theology of the University of Paris . . .
[was] usually supported by the conservative Parlement of
Paris. . . . [Together] they furiously attacked all innovators,
often with success. Burning at the stake was not infre-
quent."[15] Despite the fact that the church was firmly opposed
to dissections of human cadavers (they were actually for-
bidden in Paris),[16] Rabelais daringly performed such dis-

sections. In 1537, in fact, six years before the great anatomist Andreas Vesalius would publish *De humani corporis fabrica*, Rabelais began his summer course at the Montpellier Faculty of Medicine by publicly dissecting the corpse of a hanged man and accompanying his dissection with a scientific explanation. We know about this from a Latin poem by Rabelais's friend, Étienne Dolet (who was burned at the stake in 1546 for heresy, "mainly for translating . . . [a work] in which the immortality of the soul is denied").[17]

In Dolet's poem, the cadaver dissected by Rabelais speaks, saying how fortunate he is to be dissected publicly because "a most learned physician" (*"medicus doctissimus"*) explains to the "crowded audience" how "beautifully, and skillfully, and with what order Nature made the body of man." For all these reasons, the cadaver concludes, instead of being "food for the fierce crows, and a plaything for the blasts of the winds," he overflows "with glory" and "with honors" (*"circumfluoque / Jam gloria,"* "*Honoribus circumfluo*").[18]

Rabelais's daring dissections of cadavers and probings into the mysteries of human anatomy overflow into his art but in a strange way: through grotesque or comically obscene humor. This kind of humor—which recalls in some ways that last day of anatomy class—seeks at once to amuse and to shock. In so doing, it deflects the reader's emotions from feelings of pain or sympathy to a stance of desensitized distance. This is evident in several of Rabelais's battle scenes, where the doctor-writer obviously delights in describing the parts of human anatomy severed by the sword. For example, Friar John of the Hashes knocked one enemy's

> head into pieces along the lamboidal suture. . . . [Other enemies] Friar John impaled up the arse with his staff. . . . [He] showed his muscular strength by running . . . [some people] through the chest by way of the mediastine to the heart. . . . Others he struck on the ballocks and pierced their bum-gut. It was, believe me, the most hideous spectacle that ever was seen.[19]

Should one cry or laugh at the sight of a cadaver? Both, Rabelais suggests. We laugh at Friar John's battle-dissections, but we also realize, with the doctor-writer, that this was "the most hideous spectacle that ever was seen." Ambivalent impressions strike the reader: the horror of war along with the anatomy of dismembered, disemboweled corpses, but also the grotesque, obscene, and fantastic flights of imagination that take off from the cadaver. The horrible is wed to the humorous, the real to the fantastic. Because of these ambivalent joinings, horror becomes a ground for laughter and the real becomes unreal or ridiculous. The reader is both shocked and amused, horrified and heartened; in other words, the reader is sensitized and desensitized, pained and anesthetized, burdened and relieved. As a result of the laughter that Rabelais's grotesque humor generates, desensitization, numbness, and relief prevail. We laugh at what—when seen in normal, rather than in grotesque, terms—might make us quake or cry.

The same question—should one laugh or cry at the sight of a cadaver?—is posed in another way by Gargantua when his wife, Badebec, also a giant, dies giving birth to their giant son, Pantagruel. In reality, what can be sadder than a woman dying in childbirth? Appropriately, then, Gargantua begins by mourning for his wife. Even as he grieves, however, his thoughts turn into comically grotesque and obscene images because, as he starts to think about what he will miss in Badebec, his ideas center on her sex. Since Badebec was a giant, the proportions of her "cunt" are enormous and therefore ludicrous.

> "Shall I weep?" said . . . [Gargantua]. "Yes. Why then? Because my wife who was so good is dead. . . . This is a loss beyond all calculation! O my God, . . . why didst Thou not send death to me before sending it to her? For to live without her is no more than a lingering death. Ah, Badebec, my sweet, my darling, my little . . . [cunt] [*mon petit con*]—hers was a good three acres and two roods in size for all that—my tenderling, . . . never shall I see you again.[20]

The grotesque humor here springs from tragedy. It reminds us, too, that along with being mind, spirit, and soul, human beings are flesh and blood. Thus, Gargantua brings us back to the corporeal and earthy. Further, by centering on the reproductive organs, Gargantua's images divert his thoughts—and ours—from Badebec's cadaver and turn them instead toward thoughts of life, laughter, and virility.

Very soon after this meditation, Gargantua's fears about his own death surface. When they do, he decides that he must live and not mourn since he also will die some day, perhaps even soon. Now he must rejoice in his son's new life. Seen in this light, the grotesque in Rabelais—and probably elsewhere, as on that last day of anatomy class—is often an earthy, human defense against the fear of death.

When confronting death, disease, and the cadaver, we have seen, Rabelais sought relief in a kind of medicinal laughter that could soothe grief and help heal the spirit, soul, and body. His laughter is highly ambivalent, expressing both sorrow and joy, tragedy and comedy, fear and the conquest of fear, a vision of death and a vision of life. By means of his ambivalent humor, terrifying things—including death and the cadaver—become comically grotesque, ridiculous, and thus unworthy of being feared. In the comic grotesque, therefore, we note—and welcome—the defeat of fear.

Because we also wanted some more modern insights, we turned to two twentieth-century physician-writers, Gottfried Benn and Richard Selzer, for their reactions to death and the cadaver.

GOTTFRIED BENN

In many of his poems, Gottfried Benn (1886–1956) seems numbed, cold, and crudely, often offensively, clinical or grotesque. Not infrequently, the sexual in his writings appears grotesque, as in "Man and Woman Go through the Cancer Ward." A man speaks; perhaps he is the doctor himself. We feel the speaker's anxieties and anger as he describes the

patients on the cancer ward who are in the process of becoming cadavers.

> The man:
> Here in this row are wombs that have decayed,
> and in this row are breasts that have decayed.
> Bed beside stinking bed. Hourly the sisters change.
> Come, quickly lift up this coverlet.
> Look, this great mass of fat and ugly humours
> was precious to a man once, and
> meant ecstasy and home.
> Come, now look at the scars upon this breast.
> Do you feel the rosary of small soft knots?
> Feel it, no fear. The flesh yields and is numb.

The flesh this speaker calls numb is not as numb as the voice
of the poet-narrator. He continues:

> Here's one who bleeds as though from thirty bodies.
> No one has so much blood.
> They had to cut
> a child from this one, from her cancerous womb.
> They let them sleep. All day, all night.—They tell
> the newcomers: here sleep will make you well.—But
>   Sundays
> one rouses them a bit for visitors.—
> They take a little nourishment. Their backs
> are sore. You see the flies. Sometimes
> the sisters wash them. As one washes benches.—

In the last stanza, the death-absorbed narrator suddenly
reaches out through his shocking language for something
that is almost hopeful or transcendent. Envisioning these
cancer-ridden bodies as cadavers now, he imagines them
sinking into the earth and mingling, in that way, with the
larger forces of nature and of life. He begins the last stanza
rather morbidly, with the image of the grave rising about
each bed, but he ends the stanza almost lyrically, or at least
fertilely, with his vision of the "sap" that "prepares to flow"
and the voice of the earth that "calls":

> Here the grave rises up about each bed.
> And flesh is leveled down to earth. The fire
> burns out. And sap prepares to flow. Earth calls.—[21]

From the cold, clinical, ironical, and grotesque, the narrator
has moved to a vision of life and nature. Once more, the
grotesque reveals ambivalence: fear striving for the defeat
of fear; pain looking for healing; a vision of death reaching
for a vision of life.

In Benn's poem we contemplated human beings becoming corpses. In the next doctor-writer's work, we are forced
to contemplate the corpse itself.

RICHARD SELZER

In "The Corpse," Richard Selzer relates in clinical, often grotesque, detail what happens to a dead body when it is prepared for embalming or autopsy or is buried with no preparation. Each time, Selzer's language aims to shock and
grip. Often, he addresses the reader directly. You cannot escape from his words or from the image of the corpse.

When a corpse is prepared for embalming or autopsy,
Selzer writes, it is cleaned out by the suction trocar, a hollow
steel rod with a sharp tip at one end and rubber tubing at
the other. The rubber tubing is placed in the sink to empty.
Suddenly, through the surgeon-narrator's language, *you* become the cadaver lying on the table, waiting for the trocar
to pierce and empty *you*.

> A man stands by the table upon which you lie. He opens
> the faucet in the sink, steps forward, raises the trocar. It is a
> ritual spear. . . . Two inches to the left and two inches above
> your navel is the place of entry. (Feel it on yourself.) The
> technician raises this thing and aims for the spot. He must be
> strong, and his cheeks shake with the thrust. . . .
> Wound most horrible! It is a goring.[22]

Before long, Selzer says, your stomach, heart, intestines,
scrotum, and testicles are emptied. Seeking distance from

the horrors it is describing, Selzer's language—like Rabelais's and Benn's—uses clinical terms, irony, and obscene
and grotesque images that often have sexual overtones.

> The head of the trocar disappears beneath the skin.
> Deeper and deeper until the body wall is penetrated. Another
> thrust. . . .

> Look how the poker rides—high and swift and lubri-
> cious. . . . [T]he trocar is drawn . . . into the right chamber of
> the heart. . . . Thrust and pull, thrust and pull. . . .

> The heart is empty. . . . Thunk, thunk . . . : the scrotum is
> skewered, the testicles smashed, ablaze with their billion
> whiptail jots. All, all into the sink—and then to the sewer. This
> is the ultimate suck.[23]

Soon, along with some forty other corpses all suspended
in a perfect row, you are dunked into the tank of embalming
fluid. Only, for Selzer, the tank appears like a "casserole of
chow mein," and the corpses plunged therein are grotesque,
comical, and pitiful. And *you* are one of the corpses.

> Forty feet long, four wide, and seven deep is THE TANK. . . .
> It is . . . covered by domed metal, handle at the apex, like a
> casserole of chow mein. . . . Above the fluid, a center rod . . .
> suspends [the bodies] . . . in a perfect row; forty soldiers
> standing in the bath. . . . Upon each head, worn with a certain
> nonchalance, are the tongs, the headdress of this terrible
> tribe. . . . Each set of tongs is . . . hung from the center rod by
> a pulley. In this way the bodies can be skimmed back and
> forth during the process. . . .

> We end skin overcoats on a rack.

> A slow current catches the brine and your body sways ever
> so slightly, keeping time.[24]

Are you repelled by this preserving process used for both
embalming and autopsy? The doctor offers you another
choice. You may be buried in the ground as you are. Only,
he warns:

Now you are meat, meat at room temperature.... There is to be a feast.... The guests have already arrived, numberless bacteria that had, in life, dwelt in saprophytic harmony with their host. Their turn now! Charged, they press against the membrane barriers,... devouring, belching gas—a gas that puffs eyelids, cheeks, abdomen into bladders of murderous vapor.... Your swollen belly bursts.... You are becoming gravy. Arriving for the banquet late,... and all the more ravenous for it, are the twin sisters Calliphora and Lucilia, the omnipresent greenbottle flies....[25]

Considering Selzer's depictions of what happens to a corpse when it is embalmed or when it putrefies in the earth, it is not surprising that he envisions some other, more uplifting, end for his own cadaver. What does he wish for himself?

"I want ... to be buried—unembalmed and unboxed—at the foot of a tree. Soon I melt and seep into the ground, to be drawn up by the roots. Straight to the top, strung in the crown, answering the air. There would be the singing of birds, the applause of wings."[26]

Even though Selzer waxes poetical here as he imagines his body joining with nature and achieving thereby a kind of lyrical and spiritual glory, we cannot forget, as this surgeon himself taught us, that if he is to be thus buried at the foot of a tree, his body will putrefy and become, before it attains to the treetop, a feast for bacteria, insects, and worms. Still, Selzer's lyrical vision offers him—and us—an escape from the clinical, grotesque realities he has so vividly impressed on us. What is more, his romantic words describing his joining with nature recall, in some ways, Benn's final images of sap and earth in his poem that until then had been clinical, grotesque, and ironic. Both Benn and Selzer, therefore, seem to be reaching through the image of the cadaver toward a vision of transcendence or at least of life. And Rabelais, through his grotesque and often obscene humor, did the same.

REFLECTIONS

In the literary and artistic depictions of cadavers, the omnipresence of the grotesque and of responses revealing both sensitization and desensitization is striking. Just because one is sensitized—sensitive and/or susceptible—to death and the cadaver, one seeks to become desensitized, as though nonreactive, anesthetized, or numbed to them. Gross or obscene humor or language can therefore be seen as attempts to counteract, overcome, or blot out the horrible things one sees and comes to know.

Is it so strange that the medical students in anatomy class, like the three doctor-writers, used gross and grotesque language or humor in the face of death and the cadaver? After all, the art of medicine is a difficult, trying one, often depressing and exhausting, not only physically and mentally but also emotionally. It is an art based on, and always harking back to, the human being and the cadaver, that is, to the delicate balance between life and death and to the equally delicate balance between man's spiritual-emotional side and his earthy-physiological nature. In fact, Rabelais wrote, at once humorously and seriously, that his giant Pantagruel once thought about studying medicine but decided not to because "the profession was far too wearying, besides being melancholy, and . . . physicians smelt of the suppository, like old devils."[27] Yet is not Rabelais's humor here—and by extension, other grotesque humor—one way of trying to combat the "melancholy" aspects of the physician's "wearying" and in many senses not-so-sweet profession?

It is likely that the medical students' laughter and gross behavior on their last day of anatomy class masked, or sought to mask or defend against, myriad fears and anxieties. It is also likely that the students' reactions were desensitized, gross, and grotesque just because they themselves were deeply sensitized to death and the cadaver. And so, those students—and countless other apprentices in anatomy classes—might say, echoing Villon's unforgettable cadavers,

"Human brothers . . . / Do not harden your hearts against us." For are you absolutely certain that you would have acted otherwise when forced to contemplate, let alone dissect, a cadaver, the undeniable image of each person's fate?

3

"BUT WHAT IF SHE SHOULD DIE?"

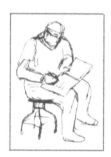

＋ ＋ ＋ ＋ ＋

> She won't die. People don't die in childbirth
> nowadays.... Yes, but what if she should die?
> —Hemingway

CASE HISTORY

It is Memorial Day on the medical wards. By late afternoon I have
already had four admissions, two to the I.C.U. I have hardly been
able to leave I.C.U. all day and have had nothing to eat since early
this morning. But the medical resident comes to tell me that I
have a transfer patient from obstetrics. He nods toward a bed.

Around 8:00 P.M. I finally get to her, my fifth admission. I go
to read her chart. Another instance of a service dumping a difficult
case onto the medical service, I think. Today is a holiday. We are

shorthanded. Why do they have to transfer her today? I pick up her bright blue chart and begin to read her history. Suddenly, I have a fearful premonition: this is not going to be an ordinary case; it is going to be a terrible one. I wish I could close the chart and walk away. The words become frightening. Is there no escaping them?

Mrs. S, twenty-nine years old, had been in perfect medical health. About nine months ago, she became pregnant with her first child. The first four months of pregnancy were uneventful.

About halfway through her pregnancy, she began to develop dyspnea (difficulty in breathing) on exertion. When her dyspnea progressed, she was admitted to a small community hospital near her hometown for a workup. Routine studies—chest X-rays and chest tomograms—were unremarkable, but her doctors found that her blood oxygen (PO_2) was in the mid-60s. (For a young person who is a nonsmoker, the PO_2 should be about 95.) After several days, her doctors discharged her with conservative treatment, without knowing the etiology of her shortness of breath.

Over the next months, Mrs. S's pregnancy progressed and her condition worsened: more shortness of breath and exhaustion, without any obvious explanation. In the eighth month of her pregnancy, Mrs. S was readmitted to the community hospital. Her PO_2 was now in the high 50s. Again, no explanation for her symptoms was found. Soon Mrs. S was almost ready to go into labor. What was more and more urgent, she was beginning to look acutely ill because of her respiratory problems.

It was then that she was transferred to the obstetrical unit of our hospital, a large university medical center. On admission, Mrs. S was already in the early stages of labor. Within twenty-four hours she gave birth to a somewhat premature but healthy infant. The actual delivery went rather smoothly. But just before, during, and immediately after delivery, Mrs. S's respiratory status deteriorated until she was short of breath even while at complete bedrest. Her every inhalation was a gasp.

Once the baby was born, an aggressive workup of the mother was begun. Because the chest X rays revealed nothing, a cardiologist was called in for a catheterization. To everyone's surprise and dismay, the cardiac catheterization revealed the diagnosis: primary pulmonary hypertension. The pulmonary pressures mea-

sured about six times greater than normal, indicating that Mrs. S
was probably in an advanced stage of the disease.

Now the diagnosis is on her chart. It cannot be erased from
her history or from her life. Dark thoughts burn through my brain.
I am no longer tired. I search feverishly for facts remembered,
ideas gleaned from medical textbooks which now come chillingly
to life: a birth from the words on the page into the actuality of
Mrs. S's disease; a birth, like her baby's, that erupts into reality
and into pain. The facts I recall are these:

1. The cause of primary pulmonary hypertension is unknown.
2. The disease is uniformly fatal.
3. The most aggressive form of the disease occurs in women
   who are pregnant, who carry a child to full term and
   deliver.

Now it is well into Memorial Day night. For the first time I
approach the young woman lying on the bed in the corner of the
I.C.U. I can see what her chart has already told me: she is in great
distress. Because talking tires her out, she can barely communicate
with me. She wears an oxygen face mask.

The history I take is very brief. Already, I can tell there will
not be the bond that exists, or begins to be nurtured, between a
patient and the attending doctor—a bond often built of warmth
or trust or caring. It is sometimes a bond of hate but it is a bonding
nevertheless, a joining through touch and through mental, emotional, and even spiritual rapport. Now I rush through the physical
examination, afraid that Mrs. S will see in my actions, words, and
expression the truth about her condition. I try to comfort and
reassure her, but I do not think I can be very effective. What am
I supposed to do? What *can* I do?

Certainly, death on the medical wards is not new to me.
Throughout medical school and this internship I have seen a number of patients in tragic and terminal situations. Yet in all my past
experiences, I had always felt that I had been able to offer my
patients *something*—some sort of relief or help, if not from a
medical standpoint, at least from an emotional or supportive one.
But now I can offer nothing.

The first night I consult briefly with a cardiologist, a pulmonary specialist, and the medical resident with whom I am working

on this rotation. No one really has anything more to offer. The diagnosis has precluded that. Although we attempt to assist Mrs. S with oxygen and medication to dilate her blood vessels and lower her pressures, my impression is that there is little we can do, even for her pain.

From that night on, almost nobody talks to me about the case. Yet if I feel isolated, how much more isolated Mrs. S must feel, for no one ever visits her: not her husband or a relative. Surrounded by all the people bustling around in a six-hundred-bed hospital—doctors, nurses, technicians, other patients, other patients' visitors—Mrs. S is, except for her baby, virtually alone.

For thirty minutes every day the nurses bring the infant up from the newborn special care unit to spend time with her mother. Thirty minutes is all the time Mrs. S can be with her baby without becoming totally exhausted. It hurts and angers me to see the nurses laugh when they carry the infant, when they place her in her mother's arms. Their joyful—and what seems to me frivolous—attitude makes even more tragic what I know is to come. Even though I explain Mrs. S's condition to them, they do not seem to understand. Or do they? At least there will be thirty minutes a day of happiness.

Several times I watch the mother with her child. She appears to get a great deal of pleasure from being with her baby. For a moment she reminds me of other new mothers I have seen on the obstetrical services: smiling, enchanted with the beauty of the new life they have created, enchanted and somewhat bewildered by their new roles as mothers. As I watch Mrs. S playing with her infant, I ponder the irony of it all. The baby to whom she has given life will be the cause of her death.

Two or three days go by. The patient's PO_2 is now in the mid-40s. Mrs. S is worn out just trying to breathe. She is slowly suffocating. Consciously, I have tried to hold off the decision to put her on a respirator because it will hinder her interaction with her child. But finally I have no choice. She must be put on a respirator to survive. On the day I can no longer delay the decision, nobody can be reached—not the cardiologist, not the pulmonary specialist, not Mrs. S's husband. Intubated and hooked up to the respirator, Mrs. S becomes an orifice plugged with a pipeline into her lungs, a lifeline that is the symbol of her impending death. Before

her intubation Mrs. could barely speak. Now, with her mouth forever gagged by that fateful tube, she cannot talk at all. No longer
can she whisper to her baby or even smile at her. She can communicate now only with her hands or her eyes.

It is the night of the fourth day after Mrs. S's delivery. Once
again, the cardiologist is trying to put a catheter into her heart.
He is trying to *do something*. During the procedure, Mrs. S has a
cardiac arrest and cannot be revived.

As the cardiologist fills out the death certificate, he reads each
word as if this were the first time he had ever seen such a document, though he has filled out perhaps scores of them before.
And, in a somewhat shaky hand, he writes his own name on the
line calling for the name of the deceased.

I tear up that death certificate and write out another one.

The next morning I go downstairs to the newborn special care
unit. I want to see Mrs. S's baby. As I stand near the incubator, I
am flooded with feelings, images, and desires, with memories that
will never leave me. I try to sort out—to master—my thoughts.
First, I realize I want to take the infant home with me. As far as
I know, her father had abandoned her mother. Would he abandon
their child as well? Then I try to imagine how this little girl will
grow up. I hope she will never know the truth about her mother's
death: if she had not been born, her mother might have lived,
perhaps for many years. And somehow I begin to hope—it's not
impossible, is it?—that those visits the infant had had for thirty
minutes a day during the first three days of her life would permit
her, in some mysterious and miraculous way, to know her mother.
A few moments of love cannot be meaningless, can they?

✦ ✦ ✦ ✦ ✦

LITERARY PARALLELS

Mrs. S's doctors had given her virtually no emotional support. Because we wondered how some other doctors had
reacted when one of their patients died as a result of childbirth, we turned to literature. But literature, which is so lav-
ish in examples of loves licit and illicit, of passions healing
and destroying, and in its depictions of other rites de pas-

sage, is strangely stingy in its depictions of mothers dying as a result of pregnancy or childbirth. Why? For centuries, after all, every pregnancy ran a certain risk of maternal mortality. Then why does so little imaginative literature describe it? Is it because so much literature is written by men, and no man can fully understand the physical, emotional, and spiritual states relating to childbearing and parturition? Yet books are written by women, too. Is it because women writers are more concerned with other matters, not with what they might consider the merely mundane task of bearing babies and expelling them from the womb? These suggestions are possible. But might there be a more compelling reason: that of a taboo that has been promulgated and perpetuated in Western culture, a taboo that says one does not speak about childbirth—except in purely clinical terms or in sentimentalized, romanticized language? Still, despite this taboo, there exist some examples in literature. No taboo remains unviolated. Three nineteenth- and twentieth-century depictions are particularly apropos.

WAR AND PEACE

In Tolstoy's *War and Peace,* it is two months after the battle of Austerlitz. Prince Andrew Bolkónski, who was wounded in the battle, is presumed dead. His pregnant wife, the little princess Lise, lives at the Bolkónski country estate with her crotchety old father-in-law, Nicholas, and her sister-in-law, Princess Mary.

Immediately after breakfast one March morning, Lise's labor begins. A midwife comes. Although the family had sent for a doctor from Moscow, he has not arrived yet. An old nurse, who comes to sit with Princess Mary, tries to reassure her. "'God is merciful, doctors are never needed,' she said."[1]

Night falls. The house is hushed but no one sleeps. Suddenly there are noises and voices. Prince Andrew has come home, and with him has come the doctor: "(they had met at the last post station)," Tolstoy interpolates.[2] How important is the doctor? As described here, his arrival is incidental.

Prince Andrew enters his wife's room. We perceive Lise through her husband's eyes and conscience:

> The little princess lay supported by pillows, with a white cap on her head (the pains had just left her). Strands of black hair lay round her inflamed and perspiring cheeks.... Her glittering eyes, filled with childlike fear and excitement, rested on him without changing their expression. "I love you all and have done no harm to anyone; why must I suffer so? Help me!" her look seemed to say.... Prince Andrew ... kissed her forehead....
>
> "I expected help from you and I get none from you either!" said her eyes.

When Lise's contractions resume, the midwife tells Prince Andrew to leave the room. Within minutes there are moans, cries, and a horrible shriek.

> Piteous, helpless, animal moans came through the door. Prince Andrew got up, went to the door, and tried to open it. Someone was holding it shut.... He began pacing the room. The screaming ceased, and a few more seconds went by. Then suddenly a terrible shriek—it could not be hers, she could not scream like that—came from the bedroom. Prince Andrew ran to the door; the scream ceased and he heard the wail of an infant.
>
> "What have they taken a baby in there for?" thought Prince Andrew....
>
> Then suddenly he realized the joyful significance of that wail; tears choked him, and leaning his elbows on the window sill he began to cry, sobbing like a child.[3]

His "sobbing like a child" is at once endearing and condemning. It suggests his childlike surrender to the wonder he feels but also his egotistical self-absorption. For he has not thought about the infant's mother.

The door opened. The doctor with his short sleeves tucked up, without a coat, pale and with a trembling jaw, came out of the room. Prince Andrew turned to him, but the doctor gave him a bewildered look and passed by without a word. A woman rushed out and seeing Prince Andrew stopped, hesitating on the threshold. He went into his wife's room. She was lying dead, in the same position he had seen her in five minutes before. . . .

"I love you all, and have done no harm to anyone; and what have you done to me?"—said her charming, pathetic dead face.[4]

How does the reader feel about the doctor who offers no help to the man who has simultaneously become a father and a widower? Do we feel angry with him? Or do we understand and sympathize with his pale and "bewildered look, his trembling jaws," and his speechless state?

Throughout his depiction of Lise's labor, Tolstoy has made us feel her fear, exhaustion, and pain. Above all, he has made us aware of her isolation, which comes to weigh heavily and guiltily on us. Several times we perceive her uncomprehending and accusing words, "What have you done to me?" For example, when Prince Andrew goes to her coffin "to give her the farewell kiss," there "in the coffin was the same face, though with closed eyes. 'Ah, what have you done to me?' it still seemed to say." And Prince Andrew "felt that something gave way in his soul and that he was guilty of a sin he could neither remedy nor forget."[5] Lise's father-in-law, too, is affected but in a different way. When Nicholas Bolkónski approaches her coffin, "her face seemed to say: 'Ah, what have you done to me, and why?' And at the sight the old man turned angrily away."[6] How can this old man be angry at the dead young woman? Is he so despicable, so inhuman? His anger might also be interpreted, however, as another manifestation of guilt or as an expression of the fury and frustration one feels in the face of one's own helplessness. Were not guilt and anger some of the emotions that Mrs. S's doctors experienced but dared not voice?

A FAREWELL TO ARMS

A detached, almost clinical depiction of a woman's death in childbirth occurs at the end of Hemingway's *A Farewell to Arms.* Or at least so it appears.

Frederic Henry, the narrator, is an American who has joined the Italian army during the First World War. A lieutenant in the ambulance corps, Frederic is basically unsentimental, detached, and ironic. Rather indifferently, partly to escape from the monotony of going to whorehouses every night, he begins an affair with Catherine Barkley, an English nurse's aide he meets in Italy. When he is severely wounded, she nurses him in a hospital, continues their affair, and becomes pregnant. By then, Frederic has fallen in love with her.

When Catherine's labor begins at around 3 o'clock one morning, she and Frederic go to the local hospital. (They are living in exile in Switzerland because Frederic has deserted from the Italian army.) Although they have not married, she gives her name as Catherine Henry.

About twelve hours go by. Frederic goes out for a rather long breakfast and lunch. Catherine is wheeled into the delivery room so that the doctor can give her gas for her pains. The labor is not going well. Catherine is worrying about dying, and Frederic tries to calm her.

When Frederic is sent out of her room for a while his mind meanders into a meditation that is at once restrained and impassioned, for it opens the floodgates of his fear.

> Poor, poor, dear Cat. And this was the price you paid for sleeping together.... And what if she should die? She won't die. People don't die in childbirth nowadays. That was what all husbands thought. Yes, but what if she should die? She won't die. She's just having a bad time. The initial labor is usually protracted. She's only having a bad time.... But what if she should die? She can't die. Yes, but what if she should die? She can't, I tell you. Don't be a fool. It's just a bad time.... Yes, but what if she should die? She can't die. What reason is there for her to die? There's just a child that has to be born....

But what if she should die? She won't die. But what if she should die? She won't. She's all right. But what if she should die? She can't die. But what if she should die? Hey, what about that? What if she should die?[7]

The terrifying and obsessive question "What if she should die?" is sounded ten times, with ever-increasing frequency. As Frederic's terror mounts, even as he tries to control it, the doctor breaks in on his reveries. Might the doctor's meditations be similar to Frederic's? For he says that he ought to perform a Cesarean.

When the doctor leaves to prepare for surgery, Frederic is left with Catherine. Because she is begging for more and more relief, Frederic, who wants to *do something,* disregards the doctor's directions about how to administer gas and turns the dial on full force. He knows what he is doing is dangerous, even potentially lethal, but he does it anyway. He tells her, "'You be brave, because I can't do that all the time. It might kill you'"[8]

Although he decides not to watch the operation, Frederic does go into the gallery to watch the doctors close the incision.

I thought Catherine was dead. She looked dead. Her face was gray, the part of it that I could see. Down below, under the light, the doctor was sewing up the great long forcep-spread, thick-edged, wound. Another doctor in a mask gave the anaesthetic. Two nurses in masks handed things. It looked like a drawing of the Inquisition. I knew as I watched it I could have watched it all, but I was glad I hadn't. I do not think I could have watched them cut, but I watched the wound closed into a high welted ridge with quick skillful-looking stitches like a cobbler's, and was glad.[9]

Filled with fear, thinking that Catherine looked dead, Frederic immediately defends himself against his terror with his talent for clinical observation, which is also his compulsion. Then his poetic imagination takes over, revealing his horror, anger, and rather ironical view of life. For the birth scene does not suggest to him a sacred or transcendent experience, such as a Nativity, perhaps, or the reverential awe one feels at the biological burgeoning of new life. Instead, the scene suggests, with all its concomitant intimations of torture, injustice, and probable death, "a drawing of the Inquisition." Frederic's thoughts reveal, too, the conflicts between his machismo and his gentler side: he says he could have watched "all" of the surgery but was "glad" that he "hadn't." Then he admits that he probably could not have watched the doctors "cut."

Frederic talks with Catherine after the surgery. He does not realize, and nobody has told him yet, that their infant was stillborn. A nurse later calls him out of the room and tells him what has happened.

Soon after, Frederic goes out for supper. He stays out for a very long time. It is as though something is driving him to eat and eat and drink and drink, to concentrate compulsively on what he is eating and drinking and, in so doing, not think about what has occurred and what might yet occur. The meal scene seems boringly protracted, eerie, and compelled. For Frederic it is a form of flight—from the hospital, from Catherine, and from himself.

> I ate the ham and eggs and drank the beer. The ham and eggs were in a round dish—the ham underneath and the eggs on top. It was very hot and at the first mouthful I had to take a drink of beer to cool my mouth. I was hungry and I asked the waiter for another order. I drank several glasses of beer. I was not thinking at all but read the paper of the man opposite me. . . . When he realized I was reading the back of his paper he folded it over. I thought of asking the waiter for a paper, but I could not concentrate. . . . I ordered another beer. I was not ready to leave yet. It was too soon to go back to the hospital. I tried not to think and to be perfectly calm. . . . I drank another beer. There was quite a pile of saucers now on the table in front of me. . . . Suddenly I knew I had to get back. . . .
>
> Upstairs I met the nurse coming down the hall.

"I just called you at the hotel," she said. Something dropped inside me.

"What is wrong?"

"Mrs. Henry has had a hemorrhage."[10]

Terrors race through Frederic's mind. "Everything was gone inside of me. I did not think. I could not think. I knew she was going to die and I prayed that she would not."[11]

When Frederic enters Catherine's room, he bursts into tears at her bedside. Now, by his presence and his words, he offers Catherine whatever comfort he can. As they talk, Catherine expresses her fears, her anger about what happened, and her love. Finally, the doctor tells Frederic that he must leave the room. Catherine needs her rest.

For a long time Frederic waits in the hallway. When he is finally permitted back in, Catherine has "had one hemorrhage after another" and is unconscious. Frederic remains with her. "She was unconscious all the time, and it did not take her very long to die."[12]

A final dialogue between Frederic and the doctor takes place in the hall outside of Catherine's room. The exchange, brief and broken, is based almost entirely around negatives. In the following excerpt, the doctor speaks first:

"I know there is nothing to say. I cannot tell you—"

"No," I said. "There's nothing to say. . . ."

"It was the only thing to do," he said. "The operation proved—"

"I do not want to talk about it," I said.[13]

Immediately after this dialogue, Frederic's repressed anger translates itself into aggressive action. When a nurse tells him that he cannot go into Catherine's room, he says defiantly, "Yes, I can. . . . You get out. . . . The other one too."[14]

In Catherine's room silence reigns, as over a morgue. Now Frederic's objective, almost detached tone returns. "But after I had got them out and shut the door and turned off the light it wasn't any good. It was like saying good-by to a statue. After a while I went out and left the hospital and walked back to the hotel in the rain." These words close the novel. They seem clinical and cold. But could any words vent what Frederic is feeling now? His pain is beyond the verbal. And like his wordlessness, his apparent aloofness, calmness, and control may be understood as his attempts to keep himself from falling apart emotionally.

Still, we wonder, can literature offer more than this—a mirror in words of our own wordlessness, fears, and flights? Can a doctor-writer offer further insights or help?

LIZA OF LAMBETH

W. Somerset Maugham, who received his medical degree in 1897, actually came to grips with his art by grappling with a tale about a girl dying as a result of a miscarriage. His first novel, *Liza of Lambeth,* written when he was a medical student, was published in 1897. Its success led him to pursue writing instead of medicine as a career. This novel is also particularly poignant in terms of Maugham's own life because when he was eight, his mother died one week after giving birth to a baby who lived only one day. When he was a mature man, Maugham said that he never really recovered from the trauma of his mother's death. "When I was a small boy and unhappy I used to dream night after night that my life at school was all a dream and that I should wake to find myself at home again with my mother. Her death was a wound that fifty years have not entirely healed."[15]

Liza of Lambeth portrays the cockney-speaking slum of Lambeth, a borough of London, where girls marry young, have babies, are beaten up by their drunken husbands, and keep on having babies. Liza Kemp's mother has had thirteen children. But Liza is slightly different. A "young girl of about eighteen,"[16] she has an affair with Jim Blakeston, a married man of around forty, who is already the father of five. And Jim's wife is pregnant again.

Whenever she can, Liza slips off with Jim, even after he blackens her eye one time. Finally, Jim's wife corners Liza in the street and beats her up. Liza goes home, gets drunk with her mother, and by the next day is in the throes of a miscarriage. "Liza began to have frightful pains all over her . . . and at last, about six o'clock in the morning, she could bear it no longer, and in the anguish of labour screamed out, and woke her mother."[17]

Mrs. Kemp rushes upstairs to get help from a neighbor, Mrs. Hodges, a (self-taught) midwife, who tells Liza's mother that her daughter has had a miscarriage. She also sends someone to the hospital to get a doctor. The news shocks Mrs. Kemp, who did not even know her daughter was pregnant. She is distressed, too, because Liza is not married.

When the doctor arrives, he offers little help or hope. His brief first visit to Liza and the cockney women is barely described.

> The doctor came.
>
> "D'you think she's bad, doctor?" asked Mrs. Hodges.
>
> "I'm afraid she is rather," he answered. "I'll come in again this evening."
>
> "Oh, doctor," said Mrs. Kemp, as he was going, "could yer give me somethin' for my rheumatics? I'm a martyr to rheumatism, an' these cold days I 'ardly knows wot ter do with myself."[18]

Why is the doctor so inarticulate? Could he not offer some help to Liza or the women—if not medical, then at least emotional? Liza is conscious now and in pain. Might not a doctor's word soothe or strengthen her?

If the doctor seems uncaring in this scene, another character seems even more insensitive: Liza's mother. After all, her daughter lies dying and all Mrs. Kemp does is complain to the doctor about her own ailments. Is her brain so addled by alcohol that she is unaware of, or unmoved by, Liza's situation? Is she so wholly despicable?

By the time the doctor arrives that night, Liza is unconscious. Once again, the physician does not offer much help. In fact, his dialogue with the midwife is almost wordless. In his extreme brevity, however, the doctor conveys— to those who are listening carefully—not coldness but sadness and agitation. As in his earlier response to the midwife ("'D'you think she's bad, doctor?' . . . 'I'm afraid she is rather,' he answered"), the doctor uses the expression "I'm afraid." This phrase, an apparent politeness, also reveals his genuine anxiety.

> "Wot do yer think of 'er, doctor?" said Mrs. Hodges. . . .
>
> "I'm afraid she's very bad."
>
> "D'yer think she's goin' ter die?" she asked, dropping her voice to a whisper.
>
> "I'm afraid so!"[19]

The doctor sits down by Liza's side. Suddenly, Mrs. Kemp shows some emotion for her daughter: "she put her handkerchief to her eyes."[20]

Liza's mother and the midwife then talk. Although they speak about Liza a bit, they seem to concentrate on their own lives and problems. Yet their dialogue is very revealing about the defenses that people, especially paramedical or medical people, use; for the midwife, the paramedical person here (although unlicensed), discloses her need for them. Like a doctor or a nurse, she must face pain, suffering, and sometimes death in her work. And confronting these, she acknowledges, hurts "a very kind 'eart" and disturbs one's "peace of mind."

> "I've been very unfortunate of lite," remarked Mrs. Hodges, as she licked her lips [from the brandy they were drinking], "this mikes the second death I've 'ad in the last ten days—women, I mean, of course I don't count bibies."
>
> "Yer don't sy so."

"Of course the other one—well, she was only a prostitute, so it didn't so much matter. It ain't like another woman, is it?"

"Na, you're right."

"Still, one don't like 'em ter die, even if they are thet. One mustn't be too 'ard on 'em."

"Strikes me you've got a very kind 'eart, Mrs. 'odges," said Mrs. Kemp.

"I 'ave thet; an' I often says it 'ud be better for my peace of mind an' my business if I 'adn't. I 'ave ter go through a lot, I do; but I can say this for myself, I always gives satisfaction, an' thet's somethin' as all lidies in my line can't say."[21]

The atmosphere seems strangely, inappropriately, unemotional. But is it, really? For are not the women's words attempts to block out, by not mentioning it, the imminent tragedy? And are not their words attempts to carve out some "peace of mind" because they "'ave ter go through a lot"?

Suddenly, Liza's lover bursts in. "Jim took the girl's head in his hands, and the tears burst from his eyes. . . . They all remained silent: Liza lying stiller than ever, her breast unmoved by the feeble respiration, Jim looking at her very mournfully; the doctor grave, with his fingers on the pulse."[22] Once again, the doctor is barely responsive. His sole medical act, symbolic at once of his usefulness—and uselessness—as a doctor, for he can do nothing here to save Liza, is to keep taking her pulse.

Because she can "bear the silence no longer," the midwife speaks.

"You 'ave got 'er insured, Mrs. Kemp? . . ."

"Trust me fur thet!" replied the good lady. "I've 'ad 'er insured ever since she was born. Why, only the other dy I was sayin' ter myself thet all thet money 'ad been wisted, but you see it wasn't; yer never know yer luck you see!"[23]

The word "luck" seems horrifying, outrageous. But it turns out that what Mrs. Kemp means is that with the insurance money she will be able to give Liza "a good funeral." Her words, which seem incredibly callous or crazy, actually hide, and are meant to reveal, a real caring.

Mrs. Kemp and Mrs. Hodges then talk about funeral directors, types of caskets, and how Mrs. Kemp's husband, swollen with dropsy when he died, had had to be stuffed into his casket. Their dialogue is grotesque, comical—and pitiful.

"Suddenly a sound was heard—a loud rattle. It was from the bed and rang through the room, piercing the stillness."[24] Liza has just died. The doctor, who had been taking her pulse, places her hand on her breast. Now the women's emotions, against which they had been defending themselves until this moment, erupt: "the two women began weeping silently."

We note some similarities between the defenses used by these two illiterate women and the defenses that Mrs. S's doctors used: silence about the impending death; busyness with other things; preoccupation with the objective, nonemotional, technical, and practical. All these defenses are attempts to stay in control—or to appear to stay in control— of an uncontrollable and wrenchingly emotional situation.

LITERATURE AND LIFE

Comparing these literary cases with Mrs. S's, we see her virtual isolation mirrored in Lise's and Liza's fearful isolation. Only Catherine in *A Farewell to Arms* does not seem so terribly forsaken, and that is because her lover remained with her and talked with her.

When we turn to the families in the literary examples, we note that Lise's husband and father-in-law were no help to her during her labor and death, but their reactions afterward—guilt and anger—provide insights into her husband's mind and her father-in-law's defenses. Frederic Henry, who was helpful to Catherine, used powerful defenses to steel himself during her ordeal, which was also his ordeal. Liza Kemp's mother was also full of defenses that made her appear cold and unfeeling, but little things revealed that Mrs. Kemp *did* care and was suffering deeply in her own way. She wanted to give Liza "a good funeral," and she wept silently at the end.

The doctors in the literary selections offer several parallels to Mrs. S's doctors. In *War and Peace* and *A Farewell to Arms,* the doctors were visibly unnerved by their experiences. In *Liza of Lambeth,* however, the doctor did not seem particularly shaken by his patient's death. Was that because Liza was so poor? Or was it because Maugham chose not to portray much of the doctor's reaction? Or did Maugham—with his medical background and the terrible memory of his own mother's death as a result of childbirth—actually portray the doctor's pain? It is true that Liza's doctor did not offer Liza or her family much help, either medical or emotional. He therefore resembled the doctors portrayed by Tolstoy and Hemingway, for those doctors, like Liza's doctor, were almost speechless. But speechlessness, as Tolstoy and Hemingway illustrated, might not be a sign of callousness; it might actually be a sign of caring. It is possible, then, that the doctor in *Liza of Lambeth* might have been suffering more than it appeared. Maugham's final words about him certainly suggest that. The doctor had kept taking her pulse. When she died, "The doctor opened one of Liza's eyes and touched it, then he laid on her breast the hand he had been holding, and drew the sheet over her head."[25] He had been holding her hand, not her wrist or her pulse. The words "breast" and "hand" suggest that for this doctor Liza was not just a patient or a body to be monitored but someone much closer to him—like a friend or a relative or a lover. She was someone whose breast he might have wanted to touch, someone whose hand he might have wanted to hold. Maugham's words suggest that for this almost inarticulate doctor, Liza was not just a patient but a person for whom, and about whom, he cared.

We think back to Mrs. S's doctors. Whenever possible, they had avoided being present. They had preferred flight to facing the patient. When they were at her bedside, they

could not really talk with her. What could they say—they
and she, who could barely breathe? They were continually
preoccupied with doing technical things—drawing blood,
checking laboratory values, measuring pulmonary pressures. They were trying to *do something*. And like the doctors in at least two of the literary histories (and perhaps in
Maugham's case as well), Mrs. S's physicians had been
shaken, stunned, numbed, and speechless. They had felt
helpless, angry, and guilty, perhaps, because they could do
nothing to save their patients. Their wordlessness expressed,
and tried to suppress, their sadness and frustration. For
wordlessness is at times the most eloquent expression of
grief.

The reactions of family members in the literary parallels
help explain to some extent the doctors' reactions to Mrs.
S. Was it because Mrs. S had no family visibly present that
her doctors reacted, in a sense, like family? Or was it because the reactions of family members in the three literary
selections are the reactions of doctors as well? Because in
taking care of such a case, doctors become as intimately
involved as family.

Literature, therefore, does offer something *that is not at
all negligible:* the comfort of companionship. In their defenses and deeds, Mrs. S's physicians did not act like mons-
ters but like men—like other human beings, like other doctors, and like the women's families as portrayed in literature. They acted like other people in similar circumstances.
Such knowledge is calming, even reassuring in a way. But
is it possible to find a better, more helpful way to react, a
more positive, more constructive way to cope? Can a doctor
find something more active than the quiet consolation of
companionship?

MAURICEAU'S CASE HISTORY

A moving example comes not from literature this time but
from life and the history of medicine. It is a case history

recounted by François Mauriceau (1637–1709), the French physician whose *Treatise on the Diseases of Pregnancy and Childbirth,* first published in 1668, was "a milestone in the history of obstetrics."[26] Mauriceau, whose name is immortalized in the "Mauriceau maneuver," was able to turn the tragedy of his twenty-year-old sister's death in childbirth into a driving force to understand, to create, and to continue caring—about the woman, her baby, and his own role as a doctor.

It was very difficult for Mauriceau to relate this history. In fact, some twenty-nine years after it happened, he wrote, "the memory [of my sister's death] is so painful to me, that the ink I am using to write it down now . . . seems to me to be made of blood."[27] But he decided to tell the story "so that the public . . . might profit from it."

His sister, "who was not yet twenty-one, was eight-and-one-half months pregnant, with her fifth child." Some three days after a fall, she began bleeding profusely. A midwife was called. After the patient had bled heavily for about five hours, the midwife sent for a famous surgeon, "the most skillful of all Surgeons, who was practicing childbirth in Paris."[28] When the surgeon arrived and saw his prospective patient in that state, "he merely said that she was a dead woman" for whom "nothing could be done but to have her receive the Sacraments." Then he left, abandoning "in that deplorable condition, and without any help at all, this woman whose life and whose child's life he would undoubtedly have saved, had he delivered her at that time."

About two hours later, Mauriceau learned what had happened and rushed over to his sister's apartment. She was still bleeding abundantly. He sent a messenger to the famous surgeon begging him to return; the surgeon refused. Since Mauriceau hesitated to deliver his own sister, he then sent for another surgeon. That doctor was not at home. Finally, Mauriceau had to perform the delivery himself. But because his sister "had previously lost all her blood," she died an hour after her baby was born.[29]

Mauriceau wants the reader to draw several conclusions from this "lamentable history."[30] First, he says, a doctor should do all that he can, as soon as he can, to deliver the infant. Second, he reasons that the famous surgeon fled from this difficult case out of fear—fear that the woman might die and fear that if she did die when in his care, other women might not use him as their accoucheur. Third, Mauriceau wants the story of "this bloodstained death" to serve as a lesson and an inspiration to other doctors, to teach them what they should and should not do and what they should and should not fear.

REFLECTIONS

On the night that Mrs. S died, all of her doctors felt something give way within them, too. They never said it; they could not. They barely spoke to Mrs. S or to each other. But the cardiologist voiced, silently but fully, their feelings of frenzy, sorrow, and despair when, without realizing it, he signed his own name on the line of the death certificate calling for the name of the deceased. That name could have been, and in a sense was, all of their names—and all of our names. For anyone who so much as observes such a case cannot help but become emotionally involved in it. Even observers are as participants. Further, when doctors can do nothing medical to save or even help a patient, they become, in a way, like all other people.

The literary histories have afforded some helpful and reassuring insights. They provide what all of us, who are so fearfully isolated in time of tragedy, really need and crave: the consolation of companionship. And Mauriceau's case history, written in an "ink ... of blood," gives us—doctors and lay people alike—a fierce and forceful impetus to action: to face, and not to flee from, a woman who may be doomed to die in the act of creating new life; to face, and not to flee from, ourselves.

4

RITUAL AND THE DEATH CERTIFICATE

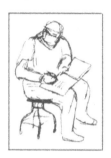

✦ ✦ ✦ ✦ ✦

CASE HISTORIES

Medical school is supposed to prepare you for your internship. During those four years you study, therefore, considerable amounts of biology, pathology, neurology and urology, gynecology, pharmacology, physiology and radiology, anatomy, surgery, biochemistry, psychiatry, orthopedics, genetics, pediatrics, and obstetrics. You are also taught a number of essential clinical skills. But you are never taught—at least I was never taught—how to pronounce a person dead. That does not really matter when you are a medical student because by law only a physician can pronounce a person dead. Interns (or other M.D.'s) thus are the ones who have to fill out death certificates. But then *you* become an intern.

An *Obolus* for Charon

My internship began the last week of June 1977. Somehow I managed to survive my first week—and so did all of my patients. Then, sometime during my second week, I was sleeping in the on-call room when I was awakened by the telephone at 2:00 or 3:00 A.M. "Dr. Peschel? Come to the medical floor immediately. We need you to pronounce someone dead."

When you are an intern and have been working for some thirty hours with no sleep, or barely any, you find it disheartening to be awakened to tend to any patient. But how much more disheartening it is to be startled out of your slumber to pronounce a patient dead.

The hospital routine for handling a death is this: as soon as a patient is discovered dead, he must be pronounced dead so that his body can be sent down to the morgue. The morgue will not—legally, cannot—accept a corpse until a doctor has pronounced it dead and has signed the death certificate. Sometimes, of course, the physician has seen a patient die, but often he has not since deaths occur in different ways on the different floors or units of the hospital. In private rooms or in rooms of two, three, or four beds, patients are neither monitored nor observed constantly. Thus, if it is late at night, when there are no visitors or routine hospital personnel around, a patient on one of the regular medical floors may die quietly, alone, and unobserved. In fact, his death may not be discovered until minutes or hours after it has occurred. Then, a nurse making rounds to take her patients' vital signs may find him. If it is clear that the patient has been dead for some time or if it had been decided by the patient, his family, and physicians not to attempt any heroic measures, no one will try to resuscitate him. Often, therefore, when an intern is summoned to the regular medical floor to pronounce a patient dead, he is not being asked to *do* something to help the patient. All he is being asked to do is pronounce the patient dead.

It is not a great role for the physician.

It was 2:00 or 3:00 A.M., then, when I was summoned to the medical floor to testify to my first death and fill out my first death certificate. Trying to clear my thoughts, I suddenly realized that during all my years of medical school there had never been any sort of formal discussion about how you are supposed to pronounce a person dead. Were there any rules, any required procedures? I tried to think. But all that came to mind was that from a medical, legal, and even religious point of view, what I was being called on to do was a highly significant act. From the legal viewpoint, this was probably the most important thing that happened in life—except, perhaps, for birth. And yet I, who had to officiate, did not have the slightest idea what specific, formal, or legal acts I was expected to perform. When I reached the medical floor, I had to ask the nurses on duty what I was supposed to do. They gave me instructions, in a general way.

I went into the patient's room. Because the body was very cold, it was clear to me that this man had been dead for some time. Coldness is, in fact, one of the best ways of determining if a person is dead. That this man was dead, I had no doubt. Still, just to be formal, I slipped my stethoscope into my ears and listened for a heartbeat. Next, I listened for some sounds of breathing. After that, I stood around for a while so it would appear that I had spent a respectable amount of time determining that the patient was dead.

When I emerged, I had to ask the nurses what to do next. They handed me the death certificate. At that point, it struck me more deeply than before that this was one of the most monumental events in life: the final rite de passage. And although I could see that everyone dealt respectfully with the dead body, I knew that the highest priority, for the nurses at any rate, was to get the body off the unit and down to the morgue. I also realized, with some guilt, that that was my priority as well, although for a different reason (I wanted to get back to bed). Thus, I saw that except in very unusual cases (e.g., a death that is unexpected or cannot be explained easily), there is very little reflection about a human life having just ended. Sitting there, holding that first death certificate in my hand, I felt somehow disappointed in the whole thing.

I took out my blue pen and started to fill out the death certificate. Since this was my first and the form is rather long, it took me some time to finish it. It was especially difficult because this patient had been admitted by another intern, and I knew his medical history only vaguely. The medical information I needed could be gleaned from his chart. But there were many other questions I could not possibly have answered. Had the deceased ever served in the armed forces? What were the names of his parents? In response to these questions and others I had to write "unknown."

As I filled out the death certificate, I thought about what an important legal document it was. After all, once it was signed the body could be laid to rest, and, potentially, the transfer of tremendous sums of money, property, and titles could begin. For a moment I felt awed by my role.

Two questions troubled me: cause of death and contributory causes. You would not think these would pose a problem for a physician, but they do. Of course, the cause of death is always attributed to the fact that the patient's heart stopped or he ceased breathing or some such elementary explanation. But when you really think about it, the cause of death is a curious question because there might be all sorts of actual causes and contributory causes: a possible drinking problem, smoking, poor medical care, lack of medical care or too much medical care, perhaps a nagging wife. Who knows? The real possible causes are endless.

Years ago, before the World Health Organization established strict rules for filling out death certificates, some physicians answered these questions quite colorfully. One old certificate read, "'Cause of death: blow on the head with an ax. Contributory cause: another man's wife.'" Now, however, the "'blow on the head with an ax' . . . would be certified as 'skull fracture with laceration of brain' . . . and as 'homicide.'"[1] How much less revealing! Or consider what another old-time doctor wrote in response to the question about the cause of death of a person who had died suddenly: "Don't know. Died without the aid of a physician."[2]

When I finally finished filling out the death certificate, I handed it to the ward secretary and began thinking about getting back to sleep. But the secretary scowled at me. "You can't use your own pen," she said. "You have to use the Brady Pen." (Brady was the name of the morgue.) Then and there, I was introduced to the Brady, or Death, Pen: a special pen with black indelible ink which was always set aside in a special place and used for filling out death certificates.

Instead of feeling angry, I actually felt relieved. Until the moment I learned about the Death Pen, filling out the death certificate had seemed like filling out just one more form—as an intern you fill out scores of forms every day. Now, this form would be decidedly, indelibly different. As the months passed and I filled out more death certificates, I began to discern in the Death Pen a wonderful symbolism. Just because that pen was obligatory and set apart, it became in my eyes an object that could guarantee, upon every signing of every death certificate, something of the solemnity and sanctity of a ritual. Such a ritual is, at a time like that, at once calming, soothing, and healing.

I do not know if the nurses sensed the symbolic significance of that pen, that it linked, in a way, the physical with the transcendent. They did know, however, that the morgue would not accept a corpse unless the death certificate had been filled out correctly: *with that pen.* And so they made sure each time that the proper ritual was carried out.

Eventually I developed a routine, very formal and very ritualistic, for pronouncing a patient dead. I would spend a certain amount of time listening for a heartbeat and breath sounds, then I would move to the death certificate. Somehow, however, it was always the use of the Death Pen that gave the entire procedure added meaning and moment.

As soon as a death certificate was completed, an attendant was called to take the body to the morgue. But he would absolutely refuse to accept a body unless it could present its proper coin of passage: the death certificate filled out with the Death Pen. Once the attendant had received that—like Charon receiving his *obolus*—he would ferry the body from the land of the living to the land of the dead. Only in that way could a corpse gain entrance to the Underworld of our hospital, the morgue.

Halloween

Over the next three years, I completed numerous death certificates and grew comfortable with my ritual. But one time I could not perform it, and the memory of that breach stays with me still.

For several months I had been treating Mr. Q, a sixty-four-year-old laborer, for a very advanced cancer of the tongue. He had done well for a while after his radiation treatments but then had begun to deteriorate rapidly. We admitted him to the hospital to give him nutritional support. Further tests revealed that his cancer had metastasized to his bones and lungs.

When we had done everything we could in the hospital, Mr. Q said that he wanted to leave. He knew he was dying, and he wanted to die in his own home. Because his wife also wanted that, we discharged him. Every day a visiting nurse went to Mr. Q's house to make sure he had enough pain medication. From time to time I also went there to see how he was doing and if he needed anything.

The sickbed was in the living room. Mrs. Q had made the couch into a bed so that her husband would not have to climb the stairs.

On one of my visits it was clear to me that Mr. Q would not live much longer. I told Mrs. Q, and she asked me what she would have to do when her husband died. She said she did not want to have to take his body to the hospital just so that a doctor could pronounce him dead. Because I knew Mr. Q very well and knew what his wishes were, I said I would go to his home to pronounce him dead, whenever he died.

On the morning of October 31, Mrs. Q called me at the hospital to say that her husband was doing very badly. I promised I would stop by on my way home. When I arrived, I saw that it was just a matter of hours. I told Mrs. Q to call me when the time came.

That night, colorfully clad trick-or-treaters streamed to our house. Every time I opened the door, cold winds, along with greedy little goblins, ghosts, and ghouls, rushed in. Amid all that merriment, mischief, and mystery, the telephone rang. It was Mrs. Q. Mr. Q had just died.

I got into my car quickly and drove to Mr. Q's house. Although it was dark outside, here and there streetlights and lights from houses illuminated straggling processions of trick-or-treaters making their rounds. Mr. Q was stretched out on the sofa, and like the masquerading goblins I had just seen outside, he too wore a sheet over his head.

I pronounced him dead in his living room. I quickly took out the death certificate because I was actually looking forward to the calming, healing effect of my little ritual. Suddenly, however, I realized that I did not have the proper pen with me. I had no choice then but to fill out Mr. Q's death certificate with my own pen. Luckily, it had black ink. But was it indelible?

I felt almost guilty as I filled out the form. For aside from my very first death certificate—the one I had filled out with my blue-inked pen and then had had to discard immediately—Mr. Q's death certificate was the only one I had ever filled out with anything but the Death Pen. Did Mrs. Q notice? I do not think so, because she called the undertakers as soon as I had finished and they accepted the corpse without hesitation. (Of course, I did not tell them what I had done.)

Now, when Halloween comes, I find myself thinking about that night. In fact, I have always felt there is something unfinished about that death certificate, something as yet unsettled, some loose end dangling.

+ + + + +

ANTHROPOLOGY AND RITUAL

Why did the doctor find so much comfort in his little ritual? And why did he still feel disturbed because he had failed to perform it one time? Anthropology offers some insights into the role of ritual in primitive cultures—and our own.

Anthropologists frequently write about the anxiety-reducing effects of ritual for a primitive people and, by extension, for ourselves. "There is . . . evidence from our own society that when ritual tradition is weak, men will invent ritual when they feel anxiety," wrote George C. Homans.[3]

The origin of the word is illuminating. Related to "rite" and to the Latin *ritus* (a religious custom, usage, ceremony, or rite), ritual is a formal system of solemn acts, religious or otherwise, established by rule or by custom. Because it is formalized as well as solemn and/or sacred, ritual symbolically links man with something beyond himself: with other men or times or with certain ideas or with the transcendent. Ritual is probably understood best in terms of what anthropologists call the "symbolic principle."

> Those realms of behavior and of experience which man finds beyond rational and technological control he feels are capable of manipulation through symbols. Both myth and ritual are symbolical procedures. . . . [While] myth is a system of word symbols, . . . ritual is a system of object and act symbols. Both are symbolic processes for dealing with the same type of situation in the same affective mode.[4]

Ritual seeks to manipulate and therefore to protect a person from what is threatening or unknown. In other words, ritual is a powerful defense against what cannot be seen, controlled, or foretold.

Because rituals are repeated, they make certain behavior and events predictable and expectable. In that way, they seem to protect one: they grant to the person practicing them a sense of security, familiarity, and control. Like myths, rituals "supply . . . fixed points in a world of bewildering change and disappointment," wrote Clyde Kluckhohn.

> People can count upon the repetitive nature of the phenomena. For example, in Zuni society (where rituals are highly calendrical), a man whose wife has left him or whose crops have been ruined by a torrential downpour can yet look forward to the Shalako ceremonial as something which is fixed and immutable. Similarly, the personal sorrow of the devout Christian is in some measure mitigated by anticipation of the great feast of Christmas and Easter.[5]

Besides offering the reward of repetition, ritual defends against anxiety in at least two other ways: it gives a person something to *do*, and it eliminates the dilemma of thought or choice. Not only does ritual tell a person what he should do, how he should do it, and when, but also tells him that it is the right thing to do; to perform the ritual is right, not to perform it is wrong.

But a problem arises here. Since *not* performing a ritual is regarded as "wrong," it is clear that anxiety is produced when a ritual is not performed or is not performed properly. Literature offers insights into the anxiety-reducing—and/or anxiety-producing—aspects of ritual.

LITERARY PARALLELS

The ritual of prayer can, of course, be powerful, calming, and healing. "To Mercy, Pity, Peace, and Love, / All pray in their distress; / And to these virtues of delight / Return their thankfulness," intoned William Blake in his *Songs of Innocence.*[6] "You pray in your distress and in your need. . . . / And . . . it is for your comfort," wrote the Lebanese mystic poet and artist Kahlil Gibran.[7] At times—as in John Donne's *Devotions upon Emergent Occasions* (1624)—literature actually demonstrates the soothing power of prayer in action.

JOHN DONNE

In late November 1623, Donne (1573–1631), who was Dean of St. Paul's (London) and already famous for his poems and sermons, fell gravely ill with what modern specialists have diagnosed as relapsing fever.[8] During his illness and convalescence, he wrote his *Devotions,* those impassioned outpourings about body and soul, sin and sickness, fear and hope, man and God, death and Eternal Life. The book contains twenty-three chapters, which Donne called "The Stations of the Sickness," an evident reference to the Stations of the Cross. Just as those pictorial representations of Jesus' sufferings are offered as objects for meditation and prayer, so are Donne's sufferings.

Each chapter has three parts: a "Meditation" on the human condition, an "Expostulation to God," and a "Prayer." In what has become the most famous Meditation (it inspired Hemingway's title *For Whom the Bell Tolls*), Donne found that a bell tolling for another person became for him a memento mori, warning him, with its sad and funereal sound, *"Thou must die."*

> No man is an island, entire of itself; every man is a piece of the continent, a part of the main. . . . [A]ny man's death diminishes me, because I am involved in mankind, and therefore never send to know for whom the bell tolls; it tolls for thee.[9]

The Prayer following this Meditation is at once an expression of anguish and a realization and illustration of the soothing power of the ritual itself. In it, Donne both vents and negates his anxiety. He depicts death as the price men must pay for original sin, and he portrays himself as a sick man and a sinner. Yet he says he "cannot be afraid." In fact, Donne believes that because of his prayer, his contrition for his sins, and his submission to God's will, he has received God's pardon. Therefore, unburdened and reassured, he is able to reach out and pray for the soul of the man for whom the bell was tolling.

PRAYER

O Eternal and most gracious God, . . . I humbly accept thy
voice in the sound of this sad and funeral bell. . . . As death
is the wages of sin it is due to me; as death is the end of
sickness it belongs to me; and though so disobedient a servant
as I may be afraid to die, yet to so merciful a master as thou
I cannot be afraid to come; and therefore into thy hands, O
my God, I commend my spirit. . . . And being thus, O my God,
prepared by thy correction, mellowed by thy chastisement,
and conformed to thy will by thy Spirit, having received thy
pardon for my soul, . . . I am bold, O Lord, to bend my prayers
to thee for this assistance, the voice of whose bell hath called
me to this devotion.[10]

Donne's ritual of prayer has carried him from an expression
of personal fear to expansive feelings of relief, confidence,
compassion, and love. His Meditation and Prayer are dramatic examples of the healing power of a ritual in action.

But what if a ritual is not performed or is not performed
properly? Another poem by Donne, "Holy Sonnet XIX," illustrates how the poet feels anxiety because he has not been
constant in prayer. This poem is particularly interesting for
two reasons: it describes emotional and spiritual distress in
terms of physical illness, and it contains two expressions
related to seventeenth-century medicine. "Humorous" (line
5), derived from the old physiological notion of the four
bodily humors, means changeable; "ague" (line 13) is the
archaic term for malarial fever.

Donne conveys his anxiety in this poem by lamenting
that to "vex" (i.e., trouble) him, his inconstancy in prayer
has become a habit. Even his contrition, he says, is as "humorous" and as soon forgotten as his worldly loves: he is
no more faithful to God than he is to women or to any
earthly thing. To illustrate his infidelity, the poet says that
a day ago he dared not look at heaven, but today he offers
prayers and even tries to flatter God, and tomorrow he will
quake with fear that God will punish him. Finally, he compares his sudden bursts of prayer—his "devout fits," as he

disparagingly calls them—to a "fantastic [i.e., capricious] ague."

> Oh, to vex me, contraries meet in one:
> Inconstancy unnaturally hath begot
> A constant habit; that when I would not
> I change in vows, and in devotion.
> As humorous is my contrition
> As my profane love, and as soon forgot:
> ....
> I durst not view heaven yesterday; and today
> In prayers, and flattering speeches I court God:
> Tomorrow I quake with true fear of his rod.
> So my devout fits come and go away
> Like a fantastic ague: save that here
> Those are my best days, when I shake with fear.[11]

The only difference, Donne says, between his anxiety-induced ague and a genuine malarial fever is that with malaria the worst days are those on which one shakes with fever, whereas for him the best days are those on which he shakes "with fear" of God's wrath. For on those days he thinks wholly and contritely about God and prayer, which he has neglected.

REFLECTIONS

Anthropology helps to explain the symbolic nature of ritual. Because anthropologists have shown that rituals exist in all cultures everywhere, both literate and nonliterate, they have been able to point out that the fundamental purpose of ritual is similar everywhere: to dispel anxiety in the face of what is unnerving, threatening, or unknown. In literature, for example, in the words of Blake, Gibran, and Donne, we hear—and feel—the anxiety-reducing and/or anxiety-producing powers of ritual. These powers can be seen in the doctor's ritual of the Death Pen. Faced with the need not only to see but also to palpate and certify to man's inevitable fate, that doctor could look forward to his ritual as the devout believer might look forward to a prayer: something that is above and beyond the universe of death and disintegration, something that is always right and always there.

Yet that nagging problem remains. What about the guilt and anxiety generated when a ritual is not performed or is not performed properly? When a ritual is not performed, the "anxiety . . . has been displaced from the original situation."[12] Thus, in the case of Mr. Q, the doctor was anxious not so much because of what occasioned his ritual in the first place—the corpse or death itself—but because he had failed to perform the ritual associated with that death. And Donne experienced a malariallike malaise not because of any physical disease but because he felt he had been delinquent in his devotion to prayer.

Can one allay this anxiety? According to Homans, this kind of "secondary or displaced anxiety" can be alleviated by what he calls a *"secondary ritual"*—a "ritual of purification and expiation."[13] Donne's guilt-ridden sonnet, in which he seeks atonement through suffering, is such a ritual. Perhaps, too, by this act of writing and telling, the doctor who found relief in the ritual of the death certificate is performing a ritual of purification and expiation, that is, a kind of confession and a quest for healing. And is not the quest for healing—of the patient but also, in a sense, of the physician—at the heart of the art of medicine?

5

THE FALLEN WOMAN

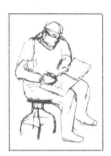

✢ ✢ ✢ ✢ ✢

REALITIES AND ROMANTICIZING

In the nineteenth century, tuberculosis was "unquestionably the greatest single cause of disease and death in the Western world," for a great outbreak had occurred following the Industrial Revolution.[1] Pulmonary consumption was "a disease so frequent as to carry off prematurely about one-fourth of the inhabitants of Europe, and so fatal as often to deter the practitioner even from attempting a cure," wrote Thomas Young in his *Historical and Practical Treatise on Consumptive Diseases,* published in London in 1815.[2]

Often the disease killed young adults. "All the tragedy of consumption . . . and the ignorance of nineteenth-century medicine concerning its diagnosis, nature and treatment are exemplified in the story of John Keats, dead of tuberculous in 1821 at the age of twenty-five."[3] In 1818, Keats, who had once planned to become a doctor (he had completed the medical course at Guy's Hospital in London), nursed his brother, Tom, who died of tuberculosis that December. Thirteen months later, the poet himself first spat blood.

> [Seized with a high fever,] he coughed and suddenly tasted blood in his mouth. . . . He looked at the bright red spot . . . and . . . said . . . , "I know the color of that blood. It's 'arterial' blood. . . . That blood is my death warrant, I must die." . . . [His friend] ran for the surgeon, who, according to the honored medical practice of the day, bled . . . [him] from the arm, the first of the many bleedings that were to hasten his course to the grave.[4]

Along with their baleful bleedings, Keats's doctors kept him on a starvation diet because they believed that in that way they were combating the progress of the disease. The poet died after a year of their medical regimen.

The medical management of Keats's tuberculosis was not unique, unfortunately, for the nature of the disease was not uncovered until 1882, and curative medicines were not discovered until well into the twentieth century. Until 1839, in fact, the disease was called by a bewildering variety of names, including phthisis, consumption, scrofula (or the king's evil, from the old notion that a king's touch could cure it), hectic fever, and gastric fever. In that year, J. L. Schönlein, professor of medicine in Zurich, suggested that the name "tuberculosis" be used because "the tubercle was the fundamental anatomical basis of the disease."[5] In 1882, the causative organism, the tubercle bacillus, was identified by Robert Koch, and from then on, tuberculosis was understood to be an infectious bacillary disease. But medicine as yet had no effective pharmaceutical remedies.

The most important development for the treatment of active tuberculosis occurred in 1944 with the discovery of streptomycin. Other drugs followed: para-aminosalicylic acid (PAS) in 1947, isoniazid (INH) in 1952, ethambutol

(EMB) in 1967, and rifampin (RFN) in 1972. Therapy is now very effective and easy to administer.[6]

Perhaps because so many young adults died of tuberculosis in the nineteenth century and even into the twentieth, the disease was often romanticized in literature and opera. It was depicted as an affliction that made people more interesting or sensitive. A prime example of this is Hans Castorp in Thomas Mann's *The Magic Mountain*. Or it was portrayed as an ailment that, in consuming the body, caused suffering that purified the spirit or soul. This is evident in the novel and play by Alexandre Dumas fils, both entitled *La Dame aux camélias*, which served as the inspiration for Verdi's *La Traviata*, and also in Henri Murger's novel *Scènes de la vie de bohème*, which served as the basis for Puccini's *La Bohème*. At times, tuberculosis was also idealized as an illness that could cause a painless death, such as in "Consumption," a sonnet by the American William Cullen Bryant (1794–1878).[7]

All these romanticized notions about tuberculosis are present in Verdi's opera *La Traviata* (The Fallen Woman), which was first performed at La Fenice in Venice in 1853.

LITERATURE AND TUBERCULOSIS: *LA TRAVIATA*

Nowhere, perhaps, is death by tuberculosis more lyrically romanticized than in *La Traviata*. As the opera opens, Violetta Valery, a beautiful, young, and consumptive courtesan—La Traviata or The Fallen Woman of the title—is giving a nightlong party. A short while before, however, she was bedridden as a result of her disease. When asked if she can really enjoy herself now, Violetta says that she places her faith in "pleasure" because "with that medicine" (*con tal farmaco*), she is used to soothing her "ills" (*i mali sopir*).[8]

At her party, Violetta is introduced to Alfredo Germont, a young man who, she learns, came to inquire about her every day when she was ill. Violetta at first makes light of this information. Later she will remember and be moved by it.

Violetta's illness soon makes its dramatic appearance. Just as she invites her guests to go into the next room to dance, she turns pale. Violetta tries to deny her illness when her friends ask her what is wrong, but she feels faint and must sit down. Admitting that she is trembling, she tells her guests to dance without her. All—except Alfredo—obey.

Thinking she is alone, Violetta looks in the mirror and confronts her illness. "Oh, what pallor!" she exclaims. Suddenly, she notices Alfredo. He asks if she is feeling better and then blurts out that her life-style is killing her, that if she were his, he would watch over her because he has loved her for a whole year. Not insensitive to Alfredo's protestations of love and his obvious anxiety about her health, Violetta tells him that he may return the next day.

At dawn Violetta's guests depart. When she is alone, she sings her splendid arias "Ah, fors'è lui . . ." and "Sempre libera. . . ." Here she begins to reveal the conflicts within herself, between the courtesan whose medicine for all her ills was pleasure and the soul within her which longs to be loved and loving. After asking herself if she can disdain love for what she condemns as the "sterile follies" of her courtesan's life-style, Violetta glides into a romantic reverie ("Ah, fors'è lui . . .") in which she thinks about Alfredo, her dreams, and her illness. Suddenly, in a strange metaphor, she links her tuberculosis with her images of Alfredo and love. Recalling how Alfredo came to inquire about her daily when she was ill, she transforms her memories of her tubercular fever into the metaphoric "new fever" of love.

> Ah, perhaps he's the one my soul,
> lonely amid these tumults,
> took joy in painting frequently
> with its hues of mystery.
> He, who meek and vigilant
> came by my sickroom door above,

and kindled a new fever
rousing me to love![9]

After dreaming like this for a while, Violetta stops herself
short, and the counterpoint of the courtesan's claims begins.
Rejecting her romantic reveries as "madness" and "delirium," the woman who must earn her living as a courtesan
assesses her real situation in Paris.

What madness! A vain delirium in this!
Poor woman, lonely, abandoned
in this populous wilderness
people call Paris,
what hope have I?
What should I do?
To joy, fly!
To die in whirls of pleasure! Of pleasure I'll die!
To joy, fly![10]

It is striking here that even when Violetta says that she
"should" pursue pleasure, images of death appear as if to
remind her of her mortal illness: "To die in whirls of pleasure! Of pleasure I'll die!"

Continuing with the courtesan's claims but even more
impassioned now, Violetta declares in her next aria
("Sempre libera . . .") that she "must" go "from joy to joy"
and that "to ever new delights" her thoughts "must fly." The
word "must," which is repeated, implies obligation, compulsion, or necessity. Violetta seems to be trying to convince
herself that she *has* to continue her courtesan's life-style.
Once more as in "Ah, fors'è lui . . . ," an image of death
("let day die") insinuates itself into her apparently (but only
apparently) joyful resolution to pursue pleasure at all costs.

I must frolic always free
from joy to joy;
I want my life to seek
the paths of pleasure.
Let dawn dawn, or let day die,

> always happy at parties am I,
> and to ever new delights
> my thoughts must fly.[11]

With these words, Act I ends. Although Violetta appears to be saying that she will, because she *must,* continue her courtesan's life-style, her words actually reveal her longing for the opposite. In fact, we sense the conflict between the courtesan Violetta has been and the loving woman she will become, even while she seems to be voicing most strongly her courtesan's claims. Why *must* Violetta pursue her courtesan life-style? She is trying to force herself to flee from what she really craves: love.

What is the role of tuberculosis in Violetta's development so far? It is probably accurate to say that Violetta was drawn to Alfredo just because of her illness. At her party he stayed with her, showed concern for her health, and declared his love for her when she was feeling ill, and in "Ah, fors'è lui . . ." she recalls how he had inquired about her every day. There is a link, therefore, between her nascent love for Alfredo and her tuberculosis. Her disease and the knowledge of her impending death are, along with her basic nature and character, some of the most important factors that help transform her from a pleasure-seeking courtesan into a romantic and spiritualized person—a person who will show herself capable of great love and tremendous personal sacrifice.

By the beginning of Act II, Violetta has already given up everything for love. She and Alfredo have been living together in the country for three months. Suddenly, however, Alfredo's joy is shattered when he learns from her servant that to meet their expenses Violetta is selling all her possessions in Paris. Stung with shame and remorse, Alfredo rushes off to try to amass the money needed.

When Alfredo leaves, Violetta enters. She is expecting a man on business and when he arrives, she tells her servant to show him in immediately. Instead of the businessman, however, it is Giorgio Germont, Alfredo's father. The ensuing dialogue between Violetta and Germont is central to Violetta's further transformation from the romantic woman she has already become to a spiritualized one.

Germont, who has come from Provence to try to reclaim his son, angrily accuses Violetta of letting Alfredo squander all his money on her. He learns, however, that she is selling all her worldly possessions. Although puritanical and moralistic, Germont is not insensitive to this disclosure, nor to what Violetta reveals next: she has a spiritual side. For now she tells him that her past "no longer exists" because "God erased it" with her "repentance."

Germont immediately uses this information to his own advantage. Picking up on her spiritual theme, he tells Violetta he has come to ask a "sacrifice" of her. "Sacrifice" is probably the key word of the opera. Derived from the Latin *sacer*, "sacred," and *facere*, "to make," it means, literally "making sacred." It is essentially a religious concept: one gives up something valued for the sake of something with a higher claim, that is, for the sake of "making [something] sacred." The word "sacrifice" and the concept of it occur so often in the ensuing emotion-charged dialogue between Violetta and Germont as to be emblematic of it and, therefore, of the rest of the opera.

Without hesitation Germont tells Violetta of the sacrifice he wants. Drawing heavily on a religious vocabulary—with references to God, purity, an angel, and prayers—as well as on figures of family obligations and love, Germont says that God gave him a daughter who is "pure as an angel." But, he adds, the man betrothed to his daughter will not marry her unless Alfredo leaves Violetta and returns home.

Violetta says that she understands. She will leave Alfredo for some time so that the marriage may take place. But that is not enough for Germont; he demands that Violetta leave Alfredo forever. "Ah, no! Never! / No, never!" she exclaims and immediately tries to win him over with three arguments. First, she speaks of the "immense and living love" for Alfredo

that "burns" in her "breast." This figure recalls how in "Ah,
fors'è lui ..." she had transformed her tubercular fever into
the "new fever" of love. Next, she says that she has neither
friends nor family and that Alfredo has promised to be everything to her. As her final and, she hopes, most powerful
argument, Violetta speaks of her "horrible malady" and impending death.

> Don't you know that my life
> is stamped with a horrible malady?
> That I see the end is near already?
> Were I to leave Alfredo,
> ah, I would suffer so,—why
> I would rather die,
> yes, I would rather die![12]

Germont, however, remains insensitive both to Violetta's
pleas and to her fears about dying. In response, he too uses
three aruguments. She is young, he says, and will find other
men. When Violetta rejects that, he says that men are often
fickle. Finally, he resorts once more to religion and moralizing. One day when she is no longer beautiful, he tells
Violetta, boredom will set in for Alfredo and her because
their "bonds" were not "blessed" by "heaven." It is striking—
and of paramount importance to Violetta's character development—that she is shaken by this, for she responds, "It's
true, it's true!"[13] From this moment on, her transformation
into a martyr—for love, for her past, and for her tuberculosis—is sealed.

Encouraged by Violetta's concession, Germont presses
on, now offering Violetta a kind of forgiveness as well as a
promise of spiritual reward. He tells her that "God ... inspires" him to ask her to be the "guardian angel" of his
family.[14] Suddenly, Germont's victory is complete. With the
awareness of her fallen state as a woman, the knowledge
of her impending death, her feelings of guilt over her past,
and her spiritual longings all mingling in her mind, in great
sadness Violetta assesses her situation.

> Thus, for the poor woman
> who fell one day,
> all hope of rising is taken away.
> Even if God to her is merciful,
> man to her will be implacable.[15]

And so, craving love and forgiveness—from God and from man—Violetta, weeping, asks Germont to tell his "pure" daughter that she, a "victim" of misfortune, will "sacrifice" for her the one ray of good she has left in life and "then die." Twice in these few lines Violetta evokes the notion of sacrifice: she calls herself a "victim" (comparing herself, therefore, to something sacrificed in a religious rite) and she uses the verb itself.

> Tell the young girl so pretty and pure
> that there is a victim of adversity
> who has only
> one ray of good that she
> will sacrifice for her, and then die,
> and then die, and then die![16]

No longer living for a love in life, Violetta now turns to a love in renunciation, death, and spiritual consolation.

So that she will have the courage to leave Alfredo, Violetta asks Germont to embrace her as a daughter—perhaps as the pure daughter for whom she is sacrificing her love and her life. Germont, not unmoved by Violetta's sacrifice, embraces her, calls her "generous," and asks what he can do for her. Filled with thoughts of her imminent death, Violetta asks him to tell Alfredo of her "sacrifice" so that he will not curse her memory. The exchange between Germont and Violetta which follows is a lyrical outpouring of death thoughts, images of sacrifice, and promises of heavenly reward.

> VIOLETTA
> I'll die!
> So that he

won't curse my memory,
let someone tell him at least
how I suffered horribly.

GERMONT
No, generous girl, live,
and happy you should be;
one day for these tears you'll have
heaven's mercy.

VIOLETTA
Tell him the sacrifice
I made in love, for I
shall love him until
my heart's final sigh.

GERMONT
Recompense there will be
for your love's sacrifice;
of such a noble deed,
you'll be proud, you'll see,
yes, yes, yes![17]

Violetta's sacrifice suggests, above all, her spiritual longings, which are inseparable from her feelings of guilt for her
past, as well as her knowledge of her illness and approaching death. Further, acceding to Germont's wishes establishes
a sacrificial bond between Germont and Violetta—a bond
that binds both of them, each to the other. Violetta's sacrifice
thus suggests her acceptance of many of Germont's social
and religious values (purity, love and marriage, God,
heaven, and spiritual reward). It also implies her craving
for Germont's forgiveness and paternal affection, for Violetta
asks him to "embrace" her "as a daughter," and he does so.
On the other side of the bond, Germont's embracing Violetta
suggests that he is not uninvolved in her sacrifice. In the
opera's final act, in fact, it becomes clear just how strong
the sacrificial bond between Germont and Violetta really is;
there Germont's words and acts reveal how much Violetta
has been able to teach this puritanical and moralistic—but

not uncaring—man about the true meanings of charity, forgiveness, sacrifice, and love.

After Germont exits, Alfredo returns. Distressed because he has received a stern letter from his father saying that he is coming to see him, Alfredo fails to understand how distraught Violetta is. Weeping, she exclaims in a burst of self-renouncing passion, "Love me, Alfredo, / Love me as much as I love you! / Good-bye!"[18] She then rushes away.

Alfredo is left alone. Moments later a man brings a note from Violetta saying that she has left him. Germont enters and tries to convince his son to return home, but Alfredo barely listens. Consumed with anger, he exclaims that Violetta has gone to a party (given by Flora, one of her courtesan friends) and rushes out, vowing "retaliation."

That night, at Flora's party, we observe Violetta's further spiritual transformation. The gathering, the type of affair Violetta once delighted in, is replete with dancers, fortune-tellers, drinking, dining, and gambling. Alfredo enters. Soon after, Violetta enters with one of her former lovers, the Baron. When she notices Alfredo, Violetta calls on God, as she will do increasingly in this scene, for pity and help: "Have pity, dear God, have pity, / dear God, on me!"[19]

When the others go in to dinner, Violetta meets alone with Alfredo and begs him to leave. Alfredo says he will leave only if she will follow him. "Ah! no, never!" Violetta exclaims. She tells him she has made a "sacred vow" to flee from him. The word "sacred" is not lost on Alfredo, who demands to know who could have forced her to make such a vow. Violetta answers, "One who had every right." Because she does not explain herself, Alfredo assumes that it was the Baron and asks her if she loves him. Lying now to consummate her sacrifice, Violetta forces herself to say "Yes." Enraged, Alfredo calls everyone in to witness a terrible scene. When all are assembled, he tells them that Violetta has spent all her money on him and now he is paying her back. Contemptuously and contemptibly, he throws his winnings from the gaming table at her. Violetta faints.

Germont arrives and denounces his son for treating a woman so shamefully. At the same time, Germont admits to himself Violetta's virtue and fidelity to Alfredo. Alfredo, humiliated, says he despises himself for what he has done. As this powerful act closes, we hear the spiritually transformed Violetta, who has revived, saying how much love there is in her heart for Alfredo. Violetta's words here, like her music, are sublime, focusing on love, renunciation, death, and heaven.

> Alfredo, Alfredo, you cannot understand
> all the love my heart contains.
> You do not know that I have proved it even at
> the price of your disdain.
> The time will come, though, when you will know
> how much I loved you; you'll admit it, too. . . .
> May God then save you from remorse!
> Ah! when I am dead I will still love you.[20]

With Violetta's words filtering through Alfredo's and Germont's, this act ends.

As Act III opens, Violetta is dying. At 7:00 A.M., Dr. Grenvil comes to see her. Violetta tries to rise but cannot and must be helped by the doctor and her faithful servant, Annina.

The brief scene between Violetta and Dr. Grenvil is touching in its simplicity and in its disclosure about what nineteenth-century medicine could—or could not do—for tuberculosis. Dr. Grenvil takes Violetta's pulse and asks how she is feeling and if she slept well that night. When Violetta responds that she did sleep well, the doctor says, "Have courage, then, / convalescence is not far off." Violetta appreciates his encouraging words, which she calls the "white lie that doctors are permitted to use."[21] Dr. Grenvil does not deny this. He leaves, promising to return later. But Dr. Grenvil gives his true medical opinion to Annina, who has asked how Violetta really is. Because of her "phthisis," Violetta has only a few hours to live. Thus, this doctor who knows his medical limitations supports his tuberculitic patient in the only way he can—with kindness, kind words, and a "white lie" that offers hope. He also takes her pulse, thereby giving the impression that he is performing some kind of medical act (he is, although by that act he cannot help his patient here), and promises to return later. This doctor can do nothing medically but he does all he can humanly.

Violetta's thoughts are concentrated now on death and religion. She has told Dr. Grenvil that although her body is suffering, her soul is at peace. The night before she was comforted by a "pious priest," as "religion is a relief to those who suffer."

When she is alone, Violetta rereads a letter she received some time before from Germont. In it, he says that he has told Alfredo of her "sacrifice" and that Alfredo, who was abroad, is coming to ask her forgiveness. Germont, too, is on his way. But Violetta has almost given up hope. In a gesture that recalls how, during her party in Act I, when she felt ill and thought herself alone, she had looked in the mirror and was startled by her "pallor," Violetta, who is now really alone, looks in the mirror and finds herself horribly changed.

> Oh, how I am changed!
> But I should still hope, the Doctor said!
> Ah! with this illness
> all hope is dead.
> Smiling dreams of the past, adieu;
> the roses of my cheeks are already pale in hue;
> and I miss Alfredo's love for me,
> the comfort and help of a soul that's weary. . . .
> Smile on . . . the yearning of . . . the fallen woman, do;
> forgive her, and receive her, O God, with you!
> Ah! All is through!
> Now all is through.[22]

In this plaintive song, Violetta voices her contradictory longings for earthly love and heavenly love. Although she craves heaven, she regrets the "smiling dreams" of her past and

laments that "all is through." But this "fallen woman" also
wants to translate the "smiling dreams" of her past into
God's smiling on her.

Suddenly, Alfredo returns. He and Violetta, joyously embracing, sing a lyrical and spiritualized love song in which
they envision a reward for the pain they have suffered and
speak of a future when Violetta's health will "bloom anew."
In addition, they promise that they will be for each other
both breath and light: body and vision, the physical and the
spiritual. Once again, as in Violetta's song, the image of a
smile recurs, suggesting a longed-for reception that is gentle,
warm, and loving.

ALFREDO
We'll leave Paris, oh dearest one,
through life we'll go in unison;
you'll be rewarded for the pain you've gone through;
your health will bloom anew.
Breath and light you will be to me.
All the future will treat us smilingly.
....
VIOLETTA
You'll be rewarded for the pain you've gone through;
my health will bloom anew.
Breath and light you will be to me.
All the future will treat us smilingly.[23]

As they end this dreamy duet, Violetta's spiritual concerns become most important. She suddenly wants to go to
church and give thanks for Alfredo's return. Instantly, however, she turns pale and falters. She tries to deny her tuberculosis but then has to admit the truth: it is the "weakness" that comes from her "illness." Although Violetta
hurriedly sends Annina for the doctor, she realizes that if
Alfredo has not saved her by returning to her, then no one
on earth can. In agony, she voices a reproach to God.

Ah! Dear God!
to die so young!

> I, whom such pain wrung!
> To die when I could dry erelong
> the tears I wept so long!
> Ah! then it was delirium,
> my hopeful credulity!
> In vain I armed my heart,
> In vain with constancy![24]

Alfredo begs her not to despair, but Violetta knows the end is coming.

At the same time, both Alfredo's father and Dr. Grenvil arrive. Germont says he has come to embrace Violetta "as a daughter," but seeing her state, he is suddenly struck with "remorse" and exclaims, "Rash old man! I see only / now the evil / caused by me!"[25]

By this time, Violetta's thoughts have turned wholly to heaven and to spiritual concerns. Calling Alfredo to her bedside, she gives him a locket containing her picture and tells him that if a pure young virgin falls in love with him, he should marry her. She herself, she says, will be "among the angels" praying for her and for him. It is significant that Violetta does not want Alfredo to marry the kind of girl she was but the kind of girl she now wishes she could have been. It is also noteworthy that Violetta believes she has earned her heavenly reward.

> If a pure virgin
> in the flower of her youth
> gives her heart to you, . . .
> I want you to make her your wife . . . I do.
> Give her this portrait;
> tell her it's a gift from someone who
> among the angels
> is praying for her, for you.[26]

After Violetta voices her sublime renunciation, the final consummation of her sacrifice, Germont, Dr. Grenvil, and Annina say that as long as they have tears, they will weep for her. We see here how fully the sacrificial bond between

Germont and Violetta has transformed not only Violetta but also Germont. For now, in addition to feeling great remorse for the harm he did, Germont believes that Violetta will become a heavenly creature, one of the "blessèd spirits."

> GERMONT, DOCTOR, ANNINA
> As long as my eyes have tears
> I shall weep for you.
> Fly to the blessèd spirits,
> God is calling you.[27]

As though released by their words, Violetta says she no longer feels pain and, in fact, feels herself reviving.

> It's strange!
> The painful spasms have ceased!
> I feel born in me,
> stirring me, unusual strength!
> Ah! why I'm coming back to life!
> O joy![28]

She falls. Dr. Grenvil takes her pulse. She is dead.

In this final act, Violetta's martyrdom is completed. Her death by tuberculosis is romanticized, of course. Not only is it portrayed as painless but also as spiritualized, idealized, and even joyful. After all, Violetta's last words—the words of the consumptive courtesan transformed by her tuberculosis, her love, her feelings of guilt for her past, and her sacrifice—are "O joy!" The title of Verdi's opera is sublimely ironic, therefore, because "La Traviata," "The Fallen Woman," has become a spiritualized, idealized, awe-inspiring being.

✛ ✛ ✛ ✛ ✛

CASE HISTORY: THE FALLEN WOMAN

Do real people with tuberculosis behave in any way like Violetta?

I recall one unforgettable case I treated—unforgettable because it was a very difficult case; because it taught me a lot about tuberculosis, illness, and romanticizing; and because it could also be called, for very different, but also ironic, reasons, The Fallen Woman.

During a whole lifetime as a physician, certain cases stand out when you know that your particular medical management has played a crucial role in determining whether a patient has lived or died. I had one such case when I was an intern.

When Mrs. T, age sixty-five, was admitted to my service, she did not seem like a very interesting case. Because she had a slight cardiac arrhythmia, she was admitted to the C.C.U. During her workup, however, we learned that she had numerous other medical problems. Since she had an abnormal chest X ray and had been suffering from fevers and weight loss, we suspected a diagnosis of tuberculosis, which we subsequently documented.

We started her on the conventional triple therapy (three different antibiotics) while she was in the hospital. Instead of improving after the first week, however, Mrs. T got worse. We discovered that she was having a relatively rare and unusually severe toxic reaction to the antibiotics, which had produced liver necrosis. It was probably one of the worst cases our hospital, a major university teaching center, had ever seen.

The sequence of events was like a nightmare. First, Mrs. T went into hepatic failure, which led to kidney failure, respiratory failure, and a very puzzling type of autoimmune problem that prevented us from giving her any transfusions. She also developed secondary infections. Naturally, we had to put her in the I.C.U. and on a respirator. At one time or another, almost every major organ system in her body went into failure, and we had to call in virtually every subspecialty in the hospital to consult on her case.

Since we knew that all her problems were idiosyncratic and iatrogenic, we had the feeling that everything was reversible, if only we could get her over each acute insult or crisis. But she was such a metabolic and immunologic disaster that every day a new—and life-threatening—crisis would occur.

Because Mrs. T. was my patient and because her case was so complicated, I was actually the only doctor who could keep track of all that was happening to her. The nights I was on call, in addition to admitting all new patients and taking care of all my other patients plus all the other interns' patients (when those interns had gone home), I had to stay up through the night trying to get Mrs. T stabilized. And the nights I was not on call I would often stay late to make sure that all her tests had been done so that she would be stable enough to get through the night when another intern, who would not know *all* her problems, was covering for me. Needless to say, it was an unbelievable struggle to keep her alive. At one point, her problem list included respiratory failure, cardiac arrhythmias, bleeding from a gastric ulcer, possible small bowel obstruction, liver failure, renal failure, pleural effusion, hemolytic anemia, a bleeding disorder, and possible meningitis. And that was when things were not too bad.

Mrs. T was in the I.C.U. for about two months. On at least three occasions, I had called members of her family to inform them that I thought her death was imminent and to suggest they might want to come in and be with her.

Finally, things slowly began to reverse themselves one by one, and Mrs. T began to recover. I think that all the doctors who participated in her care felt this was one instance where virtually tireless, obsessive work plus modern medical technology had been able to pull a patient from death. Of course, I had a tremendous emotional investment in this patient, even though I did not really know her. After all, she had been conscious only during her first week in the hospital. Subsequently, with all her catastrophic complications, she had been semicomatose or unconscious most of the time. In addition, she had been hooked up to a respirator; that, of course, prevented her from speaking. I really had no idea, therefore, what kind of person she was. But I did begin to realize as she improved, became more alert, and was taken off the respirator, that she was not very bright or particularly pleasant. In fact, the more conscious she became, the less I liked her. But I put that out of my mind.

When almost all of Mrs. T's problems reversed themselves, she was transferred from the I.C.U. to the regular medical floor. By then, I had rotated to another service, but I still checked up on her from time to time to see how she was doing.

When Mrs. T was ready to be discharged, she was scheduled for my outpatient clinic since she was really my patient. I was to see her in about three weeks. I looked with great fondness on Mrs. T's case because of the tremendous amount of time, effort, and energy I had put into it and because I presented it at Grand Rounds, where there was a tremendous amount of interest in it. It was, in fact, a memorable case for everyone.

The week finally came when Mrs. T was to see me in my outpatient clinic. The doctors in Infectious Diseases had been seeing her regularly because she was on secondary tuberculosis drugs, and I had heard from them that she was doing fantastically well.

The day of her appointment I got a message that Mrs. T was calling me. I imagined that it was probably to confirm her appointment with "The Wonderful Doctor Who Had Saved Her Life." I answered the telephone in a kind of joyous tone, only to find that Mrs. T was canceling her appointment because, she said, "There's a bit of snow on the ground and it's too much trouble to go out and get into the cab." Trying to be helpful, I said, "We could make the appointment another time," but she answered, "I don't see why I have to see any more doctors. I'm feeling fine now."

I hung up in disbelief. This great case of mine, this woman whose life I had been instrumental in saving, had absolutely no understanding or appreciation of what had happened or of what my role had been in her care. Far from being a symbol of the Great Healer, I was, in her eyes, some kind of annoyance.

It was a lesson I did not soon forget.

✢ ✢ ✢ ✢ ✢

REFLECTIONS

What had gone wrong? Of course, it is obvious that the doctor had romanticized his tubercular patient, expecting her to understand all he had done for her. But during most of the time he had taken care of her, Mrs. T had been hooked up to a respirator, semicomatose or unconscious. After her telephone call, she seemed to fall greatly in his eyes. Thus she became for him—ironically, of course—The Fallen Woman. But his patient only fell in his eyes because the physician himself had exalted her, expecting her to be more than she really was: an ordinary, not particularly pleasant or intelligent, person who happened to have tuberculosis. And tuberculosis, like any other disease, does not make a person kinder, smarter, more sensitive, or more spiritual than one naturally is. Tuberculosis, like any other illness, just makes one sick. If that person is naturally sensitive, perceptive, kind, or understanding, he or she will probably show these qualities during the illness and after. And if a person is naturally unresponsive, ordinary, or cantankerous, that person, in all likelihood, will be unresponsive, ordinary, or cantankerous during his or her illness and when he or she feels better.

The important lesson, then, is: one should never romanticize a disease, or a doctor, or a patient. In his mind, of course, the doctor had romanticized his patient, and he had certainly expected her to romanticize him. In fact, he had placed both his patient and himself on a pedestal. But her phone call forever knocked her—and him—from that height. The doctor learned then—and has had it corroborated on other occasions—that a physician should never expect a patient to appreciate what he has done for him or her. Some patients will appreciate the smallest things, and others will never like the doctor anyway, no matter how much that physician may have helped them.

What should a doctor do? His job, as well as he can. That is what Dr. Grenvil did, in his own small way, in *La Traviata*. For if a doctor can help a patient—medically or emotionally or both—then the help he gives should be reward enough. And romanticizing is not only superfluous but also injurious to both the patient and the physician. The doctor had helped save Mrs. T's life. What more reward could there be?

But what about all the literature romanticizing people with tuberculosis? What about the other Fallen Woman, Violetta Valery?

While dying of tuberculosis, Violetta appeared spiritualized and idealized. In fact, however, although her knowledge of her tuberculosis and coming death certainly colored her outlook on life, these factors alone did not transform her from a "fallen woman" into the spiritualized creature she became. Far more important was something special in her own character and nature which enabled her to grow, sacrifice, and love, and in so doing, to rise to great emotional and spiritual heights.

In reality, then, tuberculosis—and all disease—should not be romanticized, nor should a doctor or a patient. And that is the lesson, both ironic and tonic, of the one—sublime—and the other—mundane—Fallen Woman.

6
ABERRANT
MEDICAL HUMOR

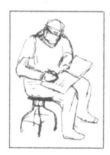

+ + + + +

There is a kind of medical humor that is, on the face of it, revolting and unprofessional. To some extent, medical sociology has noted it: in this type of humor doctors laugh at, or make fun of, their patients.[1] Certain physician-writers also use this type of humor. For instance, Rabelais sometimes delighted in describing a person's death in humorous and anatomical detail: "Gymnaste with one blow sliced him through the stomach, colon, and half the liver, so that he fell to the ground; and as he fell he threw up more than four pot-fulls of soup and, mingled with the soup, his soul."[2] Aberrant medical humor also appears in William Carlos Williams's "Jean Beicke" (a story in which the doctor-narrator sometimes ridicules, but also reveals, his great sympathy for the sick babies of poor families he had to treat during the Depression),[3] in Richard Selzer's essay "Liver,"[4] and in the title of pathologist-essayist William B. Ober's article "Can the Leper Change His Spots?"[5]

It must be emphasized that not all doctors use this type of humor. But it is noteworthy that many who do are among the most skilled of their profession as well as among the most sensitive to their patients' pains, hopes, and fears. Why do some outstanding and intensely feeling physicians at times use humor that, on the surface, is not only aberrant but also abhorrent? We turn to two instances from the wards.

CASE HISTORIES

Swollen Ankles

I was a medical intern at a large teaching hospital. On rounds every morning, our group of ten to twelve would visit all the patients on our service. This group generally included the attending physician, two residents (senior and junior), three or four interns, and three or four medical students. Invariably, the group was composed of serious, dedicated people who really cared about their patients and were very sympathetic to them.

Before going on rounds, we would meet in the doctors' room where the intern who had been on call for the past twenty-four hours would present each new patient. Our conference was private: a discussion by doctors for doctors. Because we were among colleagues, we would sometimes inject humor or light banter into our discussions. Of course, we would never have talked that way in front of our patients.

After our conference we would see each patient individually. Since this was a teaching hospital, some patients were used as teaching tools. When we visited a new patient, the intern who had admitted that patient (or perhaps one of the residents) would ask one or two questions to try to elicit crucial information to pass on to the medical students.

Dr. M, one of my fellow interns, had admitted that night. In the doctors' room he had presented, along with three other patients, Mrs. F, who had come into the Emergency Room because of severe congestive heart failure. During this presentation, Dr. M had indicated that Mrs. F was very obese, but the fact did not really register with us. Not until we saw her.

As our large contingent entered Mrs. F's room, we beheld a woman who must have weighed four hundred or five hundred pounds. She was so huge that she was spilling over the sides of the bed. In itself, such a sight would have struck us (and almost anyone) as bizarre.

We assembled around her bed. Although Mrs. F was having difficulty breathing, as part of the teaching exercise the junior resident asked her what had brought her into the Emergency Room the night before.

In a voice strangely weak for a person so huge, Mrs. F replied, "I noticed a little swelling in my ankles."

That such a thing could bother someone of her size seemed to one or two of us, at least, rather funny. With all her rolls of fat everywhere, how could she possibly have been disturbed by—or even noticed—a little swelling in her ankles?

We retired to the conference room to discuss our cases.

Dr. M was in charge. "Let's begin with the case of . . ."

"Swollen Ankles!" one of the residents said. Somehow that image elicited in our group the beginning of a ripple of laughter that grew and grew until, within moments, all twelve members of our team were roaring with laughter. We could not control ourselves.

For days after that, whenever one of us mentioned Mrs. F we would explode in laughter. For some reason, the image of that pitifully enormous lady who had noticed a little swelling in her ankles was too pathetically funny.

The Gynecology-Oncology Conference

Because I treated gynecological cancer, I went to our hospital's weekly gynecology-oncology conference. This rather large meeting was attended by about twenty people, including radiation therapists, gynecological oncologists, and pathologists from our medical school faculty, some private gynecologists from the community, residents from the departments of radiation therapy and gynecology, and several medical students. Together, we went over all the new cases of the week and decided on a mode of treatment. The general atmosphere of the conference was serious, professional, and academic. One doctor would present a case and then the physician in charge of that case would ask for the group's recommendation for treatment. Some cases were (relatively) simple and some were difficult. One case, however, was almost unbelievable. It may be summarized as follows.

Mrs. I, age fifty-three, had had a history of multiple, serious medical problems, including severe diabetes, high blood pressure, heart disease, kidney failure, and pulmonary disorders. Her medical problems made her an extremely bad risk for any kind of therapeutic intervention. She had developed a very advanced cancer of the cervix that had progressed beyond a curable stage. Because of it, she was having a lot of pain and bleeding. As if all this were not enough, there was also her social history. Her husband had died during the past year, her son had just been sent to prison for breaking into a liquor store, and her daughter had recently been hospitalized and was still sick. These additional problems were making it even more difficult to manage the patient.

As usual, after the case had been presented, the gynecologist in charge of the case asked the conference: "What do you recommend for this woman?"

There was silence as everyone reflected on this terrible story. Suddenly, one of the doctors said, "Her case sounds so bad, maybe we should just shoot her."

The whole room exploded in laughter.

✦ ✦ ✦ ✦ ✦

LITERARY PARALLELS

Why did the doctors use such horrible hospital humor? Renée Fox has noted a resemblance between medical humor and the humor of soldiers in combat.[6] Literature provides some excellent examples of war humor.

WAR AND PEACE

In Tolstoy's epic, the Russians have been retreating toward Moscow. In one battle, "tens of thousands fell."[7] By 10:00 A.M.,

> cannon balls fell more and more frequently.... But the men ... seemed not to notice this, and jokes were heard on all sides.

"A live one!" shouted a man as a whistling shell approached.

"Not this way! To the infantry!" added another, with loud laughter, seeing the shell fly past.[8]

How can there be joking and laughing in this death-charged scene? Paradoxically, it is probably the atmosphere itself that occasions the laughter, for through their laughter the soldiers try to trivialize, defy, or nullify the anxiety and anguish surrounding, and within, them. "'Are you afraid . . . ?'" Pierre Bezúkov, who had come to observe the battle, asked one of the soldiers. "'One can't help being afraid,' [the soldier said] . . . laughing."[9]

In some ways, this atmosphere of fear, pain, dying, and death recalls the hospital scene. Is it possible, then, that doctors' humor—like soldiers' humor—seeks to combat anxieties about the atmosphere of suffering, death, and dying from which one cannot escape? Can the reactions of a soldier offer insights into those of a doctor?

SOMETHING ABOUT A SOLDIER

Jacob Epp, age eighteen, the protagonist of Mark Harris's novel, is in a training camp, preparing to fight in Europe in World War II. Captain Dodd likes him, but in the excerpt below Dodd seems heartless and mean. Jacob has just received a newspaper clipping announcing that his best friend, also eighteen, has been killed in action in Italy.

And Jacob said to the Captain, My friend is dead.

Who, said the Captain.

My friend, said Jacob. Dead in a burning airplane between Salerno and Naples, Italy.

That's what happens, said Dodd, when you fly around in burning airplanes.[10]

On the surface, Dodd appears cruel. But later in the novel, Dodd, who likes and pities Jacob, helps him get a discharge from the army before Jacob is even sent abroad, whereas Dodd himself will die fighting in Europe. Dodd's insensitivity thus is only apparent, not real. In fact, his grimly ironic quip voices the opposite of what he really feels, and his humor is therefore a defense and a mask. It helps protect him from his own fear of death and conceals—although to those who understand its irony it actually reveals—his sympathy for another person.

War humor, then, like medical humor, continually jostles against death, the fear of death, or one's own feelings of sympathy. Often such humor is ironic; it pits grim wit against the grim facts. How else may the grimly humorous combat the grimly serious? There is a very thin line between them.

THE THIN RED LINE

In James Jones's novel fictionalizing the Guadalcanal campaign, semihysterical laughter, obscenity, and bravado are three ways in which grim humor combats grim reality.

Semihysterical laughter, which is akin to tears or helplessness, implies a person's lack of control over himself or over events. (We think here of the doctors' behavior in the case of "Swollen Ankles.") In Jones's novel, such laughter erupts after a confrontation with death. While debarking, the soldiers have seen one of their landing boats blown to bits by a Japanese air attack. Those who are unhurt have to march miles into the jungle to set up camp. Then they are drenched by a pouring rain. Suddenly they turn everything into a semihysterical lark.

> A hollow and pathetic lark, to be sure, when associated with the dead, dying and wounded from the air attack whom they could not forget;—but perhaps for that very reason the clowning and laughter rose to an even higher pitch, one that in the end resembled hysteria. . . . In the end, however, it did not lessen their painful new tension.[11]

Although the soldiers' clowning and laughing are described as reactions to their recent exposure to terror, horror, pain, and death, their semihysterical laughter "did not lessen their painful new tension." Grim reality is not so easily vanquished—at least not by fits of laughing.

In a way, their laughing is a kind of bravado, indecent and almost obscene. This becomes clear in the next episode. Some of the soldiers explore the jungle and come upon the bloodstained shirt of an American soldier. They hold up the death shirt, examining it nervously, curiously, and almost guiltily. Then they drop it and proceed in the jungle until they come upon a mass Japanese grave.

> It was here that the delayed emotional reaction to the death shirt caught up with them in the form of a sort of wild horseplay of bravado.... [They] pushed or poked at this or that exposed member, knocked with riflebutts this or that Japanese knee or elbow. They swaggered impudently.... They boisterously desecrated the Japanese parts, laughing loudly, each trying to outbravado the other.[12]

The key words here are "bravado" and "outbravado": they imply pretended courage or defiant confidence where there is really little or none. Bravado, therefore, explains something about war humor and—because it resembles it—medical humor.

Are the bravado of war humor and medical humor wholly horrible, unnecessary, and perverted? Or might this humor actually be helpful and even healing? A final example from literature attempts to analyze or explain, very briefly but very insightfully, why this horrible humor exists and is helpful.

ALL QUIET ON THE WESTERN FRONT

Paul Bäumer, the narrator of Erich Maria Remarque's remarkable novel, is a soldier in the German army during World War I. His company has just returned from two weeks at the front. On their last day there, 70 of their 150 men were wounded or killed. The remaining soldiers are waiting to eat.

> "Say, . . . open up the soup-kitchen," [one soldier called]. . . .
>
> [The cook said,] "You must all be there first." Tjaden grinned: "We are all here." . . .
>
> "That may do for you," . . . [the cook] said. "But where are the others?"
>
> "They won't be fed by you today. They're either in the dressing-station or pushing up daisies."[13]

Like the cook, the reader is probably startled or repelled by the soldiers' joking about their dead comrades. How can we accept—or understand—such offensive humor?

First, like the narrator, Bäumer, we should always see it in context, that is, in an atmosphere of fear, pain, dying, and death from which one cannot escape.

Second, we can understand this humor as both offensive and defensive; it is an armament, at once a weapon and a protective shield. As an offensive device, this humor causes the men using it to appear insensitive, cruel, or gross. As a defensive device, it is protective, helpful, and healing. As Bäumer explains, it keeps the men from going mad, upholds their resistance, cheers them, and gives them courage.

> The terror of the front sinks deep down when we turn our backs upon it; we make grim, coarse jests about it, when a man dies, then we say that he has nipped off his turd . . . ; that keeps us from going mad; as long as we take it that way we maintain our own resistance. . . .
>
> We have to take things as lightly as we can, . . . and nonsense stands stark and immediate beside horror. . . . [T]hat is how we hearten ourselves.[14]

Third, we can see that their offensive-defensive humor functions like an anesthetic, for in making those who use it appear insensitive, it dulls their fear and pain. There is a parallel, therefore, between the soldiers' humor and the emotional numbness that soldiers develop in battle. The most startling—and revealing—aspect of Bäumer's analysis below is that into his insightful discussion of soldiers' numbness he himself injects, when speaking of Hans Kramer's body, a typical bit of offensive-defensive war humor.

> I soon found out this much: terror can be endured so long as a man simply ducks;—but it kills, if a man thinks about it. . . . We want to live at any price; so we cannot burden ourselves with feelings which, though they might be ornamental enough in peacetime, would be out of place here. Kemmerich is dead, Haie Westhus is dying, they will have a job with Hans Kramer's body at the Judgment Day, piecing it together after a direct hit.[15]

THE BATTLEFIELD AND THE HOSPITAL

For several reasons, then, war humor is akin to medical humor. Soldiers and doctors cannot avoid facing fear, pain, dying, and death. Both groups understand that they themselves are as vulnerable as the wounded or dead around them. Of course, soldiers in combat may be wounded or killed at any moment whereas doctors tending their patients are not in imminent danger. Still, physicians cannot help but see in their patients' ills their own mortality; they cannot help but realize, like Shakespeare's Cymbeline, that "death/ Will seize the doctor too."[16]

To this grim situation from which they cannot escape, soldiers and doctors sometimes respond with a grim humor that is at once offensive and defensive. Why do they do it? A number of answers are possible.

1. This humor masks, mocks, or makes light of what one fears, including one's own vulnerability.
2. This humor makes the joke teller appear strong, insensitive, or cruel instead of weak and vulnerable.
3. This humor-armament interposes a protective shield between the object of one's fear and oneself. In that way, it keeps one from staring directly at the Medusa head of horror and death.

4. This humor is a coat of armor.
5. This humor has an anesthetic effect. It helps to mask pain, feelings, and fears with apparent numbness and insensitivity.
6. This humor pits obscenities of word and thought against the obscenities of suffering and death.
7. This is a humor of bravado, masks, and appearances which seeks to defy or deny realities that are too horrible.
8. This humor substitutes defiance for capitulation, aggressive action for surrender, courage or bravado for fear. It thus enables the soldier and doctor to defy death and fear instead of giving in to them. For example, as bombs fall on Bäumer and his company, he fires back with his wit:

> There is always plenty of amusement, the airmen see to that. There are countless fights for us to watch every day.... [S]hrapnel and high-explosives begin to drop on us. We lose eleven men in one day that way.... Two are smashed so that Tjaden remarks you could scrape them off the wall of the trench and bury them in a mess-tin.[17]

What exactly is this horrible-helpful humor used by soldiers and by doctors?

GALLOWS HUMOR

Gallows humor (in German, *Galgenhumor*) is humor with an eye always on death. Basically, it implies two things: ghoulish or macabre humor or the amused cynicism of a person facing disaster. There are excellent examples of gallows humor in *Hamlet,* Act V, scene 1, where the grave diggers, called First Clown and Second Clown, enter to dig Ophelia's grave. As they work, they talk—and jest.

> *First Clown.*   What is he that builds stronger than either the mason, the shipwright, or the carpenter?

Second Clown. The gallows-maker; for that frame outlives a thousand tenants.

First Clown. I like thy wit well. . . .

[While digging, the First Clown sings a ditty about love.]

Hamlet. Has this fellow no feeling of his business that a sings in grave-making?

Horatio. Custom hath made it in him a property of easiness.

Hamlet. 'Tis e'en so. The hand of little employment hath the daintier sense. . . .

[Hamlet addresses the grave digger who is standing in the grave he is making.]

Hamlet. Whose grave's this, sirrah?

First Clown. Mine, sir.

Hamlet. I think it be thine indeed, for thou liest in't.

First Clown. . . . For my part, I do not lie in't, yet it is mine. . . .

Hamlet. What man dost thou dig it for?

First Clown. For no man, sir.

Hamlet. What woman, then?

First Clown. For none, neither.

Hamlet. Who is to be buried in't?

First Clown. One that was a woman, sir; but rest her soul, she's dead.[18]

Watching the tragedy, we appreciate the wonderful wit of this scene, which helps relieve the mounting tension created by the deaths that have already taken place and the deaths yet to come. We note, too, the grave diggers' apparent insensitivity to death, and we echo, perhaps, Hamlet's reactions: first his shock or offense at their joking and then his realization that their occupation has numbed and thus *protected* them from feelings that are too dainty or painful.

Gallows humor, therefore, makes use of protective numbing. But is that numbness freely gotten, or is it acquired at some cost?

In "Jokes and Their Relation to the Unconscious," Freud touches on the numbing and protective—and also costly—qualities of gallows humor. He gives two examples of this humor: (1) "A rogue who was being led out to execution on a Monday remarked: 'Well, this week's beginning nicely,'" and (2) "the rogue on his way to execution asked for a scarf for his bare throat so as not to catch cold."[19] Freud continues:

> In the case of the rogue who refuses to catch cold on the way to execution we laugh heartily. The situation that ought to drive the criminal to despair might rouse intense pity in us; but that pity is inhibited because we understand that he, who is more closely concerned, makes nothing of the situation. . . . We are, as it were, infected by the rogue's indifference—though we notice that it has cost him a great expenditure of psychical work.[20]

Several things are significant here. First, instead of feeling pity, we laugh. We have exchanged a painful feeling for a happy one. Second, we understand that the rogue's apparent indifference—his protective coat of humor—has cost him "a great expenditure" of mental and emotional energy. Third, we realize that *this cost applies to other tellers of gallows humor* as well.

What do these findings about benefits and costs tell us about gallows humor, in general, and about the humor some doctors use, in particular? Are doctors different from other people who use gallows humor? Do patients sometimes use gallows humor?

In *Experiment Perilous,* Fox describes both the doctors who worked in an all-male, fifteen-bed metabolic research ward of a teaching hospital associated with a major medical school and the patients who were treated there over a period of time. Many of the patients had diseases that were not well understood and could not be effectively controlled. The doctors had to take care of these patients; they also had to experiment on them to try to devise better treatment modalities. Not infrequently, the situation was tense and/or depressing. Several patients did not respond well, and several died. What is fascinating, however, is that doctors and patients coped with this grim situation in a similar way: gallows humor.

Here is how some of the doctors talked at one of their conferences:

> *Dr. D.:* What you're doing, Bob, is evaluating these people as good merely on the basis of their not being dead, because so many of the others have died ...
>
> *Dr. C.:* Bill Pappas is a good result ...
>
> *Dr. R.:* And Walter Cousins was ...
>
> *Dr. D.:* Except now he's dead.
>
> *Dr. R.:* Well, you can't liver forever! (*Group laughter*)[21]

Of the patients, Fox notes, "Like the humor of their physicians, the humor of patients was antithetic in nature: counterphobic and inversely reverent. . . . [They] joked about things which especially disturbed or frightened them, and about those to which they were positively committed or about which they deeply cared."[22]

It is significant that both physicians and patients used the same type of humor. That is, physicians confronting pain and death are not different from other people confronting the same situations and fears. Although to an outsider the doctors' aberrant humor might seem blasphemous, coldhearted, or downright disgusting, it is—like the humor of others in the face of death—a bravado, a defense, and a means to fortify themselves against the horror and pain they feel and wish to conceal or overcome. When a doctor mocks his patients, his behavior is actually a symptom of his own distress as well as a kind of self-prescribed medicine to relieve his own pain and anxiety. Although this aberrant medical humor, like other forms of gallows humor, is macabre, it is also extremely helpful and healing. Gallows humor is, ironically, a lifeline.

SOME GRAVE CONCLUSIONS

"The closest thing to humor is tragedy," wrote James Thurber.[23] We sense this fully in gallows humor, which includes medical humor. Such humor is, of course, ambivalent. It is filled with love and hate, hope and fear, laughter and tears. It can be understood, in part, by this insight from William Blake: "Excess of sorrow laughs."[24]

Why, then, do some doctors mock their patients? They mock them because—like soldiers in combat, the patients on the metabolic research ward, Freud's rogues, the grave diggers in *Hamlet,* and innumerable others—they need to defend themselves against anxiety and anguish, fear and pain, dying and death. And they mock them because, as Mark Van Doren said,

> Wit is the only wall
> Between us and the dark.[25]

7

WHEN A DOCTOR HATES A PATIENT

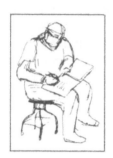

+ + + + +

CASE HISTORY: "DUCHESS"

Generally, physicians respond with a variety of emotions to their patients: some they truly like; others they do not like but still regard sympathetically because of their illnesses. In rare instances, however, a doctor actually hates a patient yet is forced to take care of him or her. That happened to me in one case when I was an intern.

Over a period of several years, one of the most infamous patients in our hospital was referred to as "Duchess," a nickname bestowed by the hospital staff. A fifty-two-year-old female who suffered from chronic kidney failure, Duchess was on peritoneal dialysis. This treatment not only demands very careful medical management by doctors but it also requires a lot of cooperation from the patients, who must monitor their diets and fluid intake. Patients on peritoneal dialysis come to the hospital to be dialyzed as outpatients several times a week. They have to become inpatients only when they get into trouble. Without dialysis, they would die within a few days.

Patients on dialysis who do not pay strict attention to their diets often require immediate hospitalization with around-the-clock dialysis and meticulous medical monitoring to correct the fluid overload and metabolic status. Since Duchess habitually broke all the rules of her diet (e.g., she would eat enormous quantities of salt), she required periodic hospitalization.

Sometime during my second month as an intern Duchess was admitted to my service. At that time, I was working in the I.C.U. Naturally, all the nurses there knew Duchess. In fact, when I was going down to the E.R. to pick her up, they all warned me that she was one of the most difficult and obnoxious patients anyone could have.

But I was not prepared for just how bad she was.

The first thing I noticed after Duchess settled into the I.C.U. was that she was chewing a big plug of tobacco and periodically spitting tobacco juice on the bed. Being naive, I asked the nurses to take her tobacco away. They told me they knew from past experience that if Duchess did not have her tobacco she would refuse to allow anyone to treat her. In fact, they said, when they had taken her tobacco away in the past, she had sat on her bed and screamed and cursed and refused to let any doctor examine or even come near her. And so, they advised me, it was necessary to bribe her with tobacco to take care of her. I therefore had to agree to let Duchess keep chewing tobacco and spitting tobacco juice on the bed so that I could examine her.

Meeting her was something less than a pleasure. Because of her fluid overload, she was in congestive heart failure and, consequently, very short of breath. Though she could barely breathe, she insisted on chewing her tobacco and firing its juice like venom or a barrage of gunfire. Examining her was all but impossible. Because she refused to cooperate, I could not listen to her lungs properly. The few times I gently tried to force her to do something, like roll onto her side, she made a fist and threatened to hit me.

Duchess would not even cooperate verbally. Whenever I asked a question, she would refuse to answer, but not because she was short of breath, for at random intervals she fired volleys of the vilest obscenities. Although initially I had felt a great sympathy for this woman and her condition, after several rounds of her obscenities I began to feel a rage within me which I had to struggle to control.

Finally, I gave up trying to examine her properly (I had done all I could) and told the I.C.U. nurses to begin her intensive peritoneal dialysis. They were very reluctant to proceed because during the past year Duchess had sent two I.C.U. nurses to the E.R.: she had bitten them and broken their skin. (An adult bite can produce a serious infection.) But they had no choice.

I came to hate taking care of this obnoxious patient. I found that the only way Duchess would let me do anything at all was if I threatened to take away her tobacco. After three days, we finally discharged her. That was about all I could stand of her anyway.

Some three weeks later, Duchess was admitted again for the same problem. On this occasion, when I was drawing blood from her, she tried to bite me. After that, she tried to pull the needle from my hand and in so doing knocked down all the samples I had already drawn. The tubes broke and blood spattered on the floor, which meant that I had to draw her blood all over again.

A few weeks later, Duchess was again admitted for the same problem. Because she was in the hospital, she had to adhere to a very low salt and fluid-restricted diet. (She was supposed to be on that kind of diet all the time.) She obviously hated her diet. When the people from the diet service came to remove her tray after each meal, she would either spit at them or hurl a fork or knife their way.

Needless to say, taking care of someone like that was very trying. My natural urges were to choke her to death. In fact, it gave me a lot of relief to fantasize how I would kill her.

Over the year, I had to minister to Duchess about four times. Each time was an indescribable ordeal of exercising patience and self-control. I had to constantly smother my rage to maintain an objective approach to her medical problems. Still, every time she was admitted to our hospital, Duchess got from all of us the best of modern medical care, which carried her through another crisis. As professionals, the doctors and nurses refused to let personal feelings interfere with the proper medical management of her case. But each one of us must have been secretly imagining her murder thousands of times over.

After my internship I never had to take care of Duchess again. About two years later, I learned from the medical house staff that she had finally died. I guess my predominant feeling was one of frustration, as though I had been thwarted in my desire for revenge.

+ + + + +

LITERARY PARALLELS

Do other doctors sometimes hate their patients? We found companionship in two American doctor-writers, William Carlos Williams and Richard Selzer.

WILLIAM CARLOS WILLIAMS

The eminent poet William Carlos Williams (1883–1963) received his M.D. from the University of Pennsylvania in 1906. Four years later, he returned to his hometown of Rutherford, New Jersey, to practice medicine—and writing. "When they ask me ... how I have for so many years continued an equal interest in medicine and the poem, I reply that they amount for me to nearly the same thing," he wrote in his *Autobiography*.[1] He stayed in active medical practice until 1951, when a stroke forced him to stop.

Williams spent part of his internship at Nursery and Child's Hospital ("Sixty-first Street and Tenth Avenue ... just across Tenth from the most notorious block in the New York criminal West Side, San Juan Hill or Hell's Kitchen, as you preferred to call it").[2] There he spent a lot of time in pediatrics. "I was fascinated by it and knew at once that that was my field," he said.[3] In his works, in fact, we sense his fascination for children, even—perhaps especially—for the most difficult and obstreperous ones. Mathilda in "The Use of Force" is such a case.

In this story, the doctor-narrator goes to the patient's house. The mother, father, and girl, "an unusually attractive little thing, and as strong as a heifer in appearance,"[4] are huddled in the kitchen for warmth. Just from looking at Mathilda the doctor knows she has a high fever. She has been sick for three days, yet has been denying that her throat hurts. The doctor and Mathilda's parents are concerned because they know there have been several cases of diphtheria in her school. But she absolutely refuses to let the doctor examine her throat. Not only that: when he moves his chair closer to her, she tries to claw his eyes and, in so doing, knocks his glasses onto the floor. It becomes a battle.

> If you don't do what the doctor says, you'll have to go to the hospital, the mother admonished her severely.
> Oh yeah? [the doctor thought.] I had to smile to myself. After all, I had already fallen in love with the savage brat.[5]

Despite his "love" for Mathilda, the doctor finally grows furious with her.

> I grasped the child's head with my left hand and tried to get the wooden tongue depressor between her teeth. She fought, with clenched teeth, desperately! But now I also had grown furious—at a child. I tried to hold myself down but I couldn't.[6]

When he finally gets the tongue depressor behind Mathilda's last teeth, she bites down so hard she reduces it to splinters. He orders the mother to give him a smooth-handled spoon.

The doctor's anger is now beyond control. Rationally, he knows that if he leaves and returns in about an hour he will probably be able to examine the girl. But he also realizes that he now relishes his anger and hate: "The worst of it was that I too had got beyond reason. I could have torn the child apart in my own fury and enjoyed it. It was a pleasure to attack her. My face was burning with it." Naturally, the physician tries to rationalize his behavior to himself: "The damned little brat must be protected against her own idiocy, one says to one's self at such times. Others must be protected against her."[7] But he knows there is more. Coupled with his fury and desire for muscular release is his shame at being defeated by a child.

> [A] blind fury, a feeling of adult shame, bred of a longing for muscular release are the operatives. One goes on to the end.
>
> In a final unreasoning assault I overpowered the child's neck and jaws. I forced the heavy silver spoon back of her teeth and down her throat until she gagged.[8]

And there he sees it: her tonsils covered with membrane, the terrible sore throat she had been hiding and denying for days.

In the end, the doctor is glad of his victory, yet he also feels compassion for the child's defeat. His final words reveal his sense of triumph as well as his sympathy for Mathilda. "She had been on the defensive before but now she attacked. Tried to get off her father's lap and fly at me while tears of defeat blinded her eyes."[9]

For several reasons, Williams' anger and hatred toward his pediatric patient do not last. First, he has conquered this seemingly unconquerable creature. Second, although he has vented his anger on her, he has the satisfaction of finding her unhealthy. Thus, the negative implications of an act potentially comparable to rape (the story's title alerts us to this hideous violation) are safely dissipated. Third, his feelings about her are ambivalent: a combination of hate and love, resentment and admiration. The doctor always reminds himself that this patient is just a child, smaller and weaker than he. And we sense that the doctor-narrator likes his patient's wildness, willfulness, and stubbornness as much as— or maybe even more than—he hates it. Perhaps it reminds him of the fierce and persistent qualities in himself, of the very fierceness and persistence that eventually enable him to conquer his patient.

What happens, however, when a doctor faces and vents his anger at a wild and powerful adult male patient? Such a full-blown fury—both the doctor's and the patient's—is described in a story by Richard Selzer.

RICHARD SELZER

Born in Troy, New York, in 1928, Richard Selzer received
his M.D. from Albany Medical College in 1953 and practiced
general surgery in New Haven, Connecticut, where he was
on the faculty of the Yale University School of Medicine. He
is the author of several books of fiction and essays that deal,
for the most part, with medicine.

"Brute" is Selzer's narrative of an event that happened
twenty-five years before in an Emergency Room of a city
hospital. It is the story of a hate-filled patient and a hate-
filled doctor, each of whom, in his own way, is the "brute"
of the title.

It is 2:00 A.M. and the surgeon-narrator is on call. He is
bone tired. The police bring in a new patient, a "huge black
man" with a gaping wound "deep to the bone" across his
entire forehead.[10] Fuming and murderous, the man seems
to the surgeon like a wild horse or some mythological beast.

> At the door, the mans rears as though to shake off the [four
> policemen] . . . who cling to his arms. . . . Again and again
> he throws his head and shoulders forward, then back, rearing,
> roaring. The policemen ride him like parasites. Had he horns
> he would gore them. . . . The man is hugely drunk—toxic,
> fuming, murderous—a great mythic beast broken loose in the
> city.[11]

After the man has been tied down on the table, the surgeon examines his wound. It will take at least two hours to
fix. Although the doctor is exhausted, he is strangely exhilarated: almost in love with the untamed man. "I am ravished by the sight of him, the raw, untreated flesh, his very
wildness which suggests less a human than a great and
beautiful animal."[12] The surgeon is "ravished"—enraptured
but also seized, as if sexually—by the man's wildness and
by the wound in which he sees not ugliness but greatness
and animallike beauty.

When the surgeon starts to cleanse and debride the
wound, the man groans, lifts his pelvis from the table, and

rolls his head from side to side. "Hold still," the surgeon says. "I cannot stitch your forehead unless you hold still." The man rages, and the surgeon-narrator remarks:

> Perhaps it is the petulance in my voice that makes him resume his struggle against all odds to be free.... But why can he not sense that I am tired? He spits and curses and rolls his head to escape from my fingers. It is a quarter to three in the morning. I have not yet begun to stitch. I lean close to him; his steam fills my nostrils. "Hold still," I say.
>
> "*You* fuckin' hold still," he says to me in a clear, fierce voice.[13]

The surgeon loses control. "Suddenly, I am in the fury with him. Somehow he has managed to capture me, to pull me inside his cage. Now we are two brutes hissing and batting at each other. But I do not fight fairly." For the surgeon explains how he takes some heavy, braided silk suture and sews it through the patient's earlobes and also through the mattress on the stretcher. Now the man's head is sewn taut onto the table, into the position the surgeon needs for stitching.

> "I have sewn your ears to the stretcher," I say. "Move, and you'll rip 'em off." And leaning close I say in a whisper, "Now *you* fuckin' hold still."
>
> I do more. I wipe the ... [clots of blood] from his eyes so that he can see. And I lean over him from the head of the table, so that my face is directly above his, upside down. And I grin. It is the cruelest grin of my life. Torturers must grin like that, beheaders and operators of racks.[14]

Vanquished, the patient stays still. From 4:00 until 5:30 A.M., the surgeon stitches. Then, he snips the silk threads from the man's earlobes and helps him to sit up. In the doctor's eyes, the patient now appears beautiful, powerful, and regal. "The bandage on his head is a white turban. A single drop of blood in each earlobe, like a ruby. He is a maharajah."[15] The police pull the man away.

It is twenty-five years later, yet the surgeon still feels guilty about that case—not for having sewn his patient's earlobes to the mattress but for his vindictive grin of triumph. "Even now, so many years later, this ancient rage of mine returns to peck among my dreams. . . . How sorry I will always be. Not being able to make it up to him for that grin."[16]

Because the surgeon was ambivalent about his patient, his terrible grin, the sign of his avenging anger, comes back to haunt him. After all, Selzer implies, although that patient felt no pity for the surgeon (or for himself), he still deserved some pity. For the doctor, who was stronger, not physically but just because he was the doctor, expressed his anger cruelly or at least unfairly. The surgeon has exchanged guilt for the hatred he expressed.

REFLECTIONS

William Carlos Williams, who felt love and hate for the fierce Mathilda, vented his anger on her and conquered her. Richard Selzer, who loved and hated his raging patient, continued to feel guilty about his act a quarter of a century later. Both these doctors could feel ambivalent or guilty about their anger precisely because they had expressed it.

The doctor in Duchess' case was different. Since he never did vent his anger on Duchess (except in his many private fantasies), he did not feel guilty for hating her and for continuing to hate her years after her death. But he did feel sad about it and wished that his recollections could be otherwise.

Naturally, Duchess' physician did—and does—feel sympathy for other people on dialysis and for other patients suffering from a variety of medical, sociological, or psychological ills. But he felt no sympathy for Duchess, who always received the best modern medical care and who always tried to disgrace, disgust, or destroy the medical staff assigned to her.

It is distasteful to think that a physician can hate a patient. But a doctor—like any other person—can sometimes, when pushed to the extreme, return hate for hate. Although it is not a praiseworthy reaction, it is perhaps an understandable one. In fact, on those rare instances when a doctor is forced to take care of a particularly abusive patient, hate may be the only refuge or defense the physician has left. On those occasions, the doctor's hate may be strangely healing because it enables him to face, not reject or refuse to treat, his patient. Still, this curiously healing hate, whether expressed toward the patient or suppressed, is itself—as hate always is—a kind of wound. It mars the physician with scars of guilt or sadness which not even many years can erase or ease from the memory.

8

SOME LESSONS FROM THE CANCER WARD

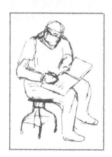

+ + + + +

CASE HISTORY

By the time Mrs. C, age forty-seven, was admitted to the hospital in early December, I had been a medical intern for five months. But in all my time on the wards, I had never met anyone like her. Here is her history.

Ten years before, after a diagnosis of breast cancer, Mrs. C had had a mastectomy. She had done well for about eight years, until her cancer had recurred. At that point, she had been given radiation therapy and chemotherapy and had done reasonably well for two more years. About one week prior to this admission she had begun to experience shortness of breath. X rays revealed a pleural effusion. She was therefore hospitalized for two reasons: because of her severe shortness of breath and because her doctor wanted to find out why there was so much fluid in her lung. He suspected that it was due to her metastatic disease.

I was the intern who admitted her. Generally, most patients do not affect an intern very much. But this woman was different. What struck me most about Mrs. C was that although she knew that she had metastatic disease, she had obviously not spent the past two years in self-pity. I learned that she was a deeply religious woman. What impressed me more, however, was that she clearly loved her family (she had a husband and children) and life itself. Her desire to continue living was so strong that she refused to let her cancer interfere with what she wanted to do.

In the days following her admission, I became attached to Mrs. C, as did some of the other doctors and the nurses. Although often tired when we went in to see her, we soon found that she would cheer *us* up and make *us* feel good.

How did she do it? With a combination of humor, spirit, and friendliness—all those "trite" human virtues that are not trite at all. Mrs. C always seemed grateful for whatever we did, no matter how small. Perhaps her faith helped her. She told us that she had one more goal in life: to spend Christmas with her family. To me that goal epitomized her. She knew she was dying, but she could focus on what was important while she was alive.

After we had withdrawn some fluid from Mrs. C's lung, we documented that, as we had suspected, the effusion was due to her breast cancer. We then called in a thoracic surgeon to put a chest tube into her lung. The tube was hooked up to a suction device that continued to draw out fluid. After some time we planned to instill a sclerosing agent in the lining of her lung. The procedure is supposed to help prevent fluid from reaccumulating after the chest tube is withdrawn. It is successful only about 50 percent of the time, but we felt it was worth a try.

The chest tube had been in Mrs. C's lung for about twelve hours when something obviously went wrong because I was suddenly summoned to her room at around 2:00 A.M. She was having trouble breathing, even while at rest in bed. We took another chest X-ray, which revealed that the fluid had reaccumulated. Mrs. C was starting to go into respiratory distress, a situation that is generally life threatening. Soon she would become exhausted just by the act of breathing.

I rushed to a telephone to consult with her attending physician. We decided that I should call the thoracic surgeon who had put the tube into her lung and ask him to come in and replace the tube. However, when I reached him at home (it was by then around 3:00 A.M.), he refused to come to the hospital. Instead, he told me to draw off the fluid myself. I was terrified. Although I had seen this procedure done before (it is called a thorocentesis), I had never done it. It involves inserting a large needle into the lung cavity and withdrawing the fluid with a syringe.

I hurried back to Mrs. C's room. In the thirty or forty minutes it had taken me to make the calls and discuss her case, she had deteriorated markedly. She was gasping for every breath now. Without some sort of intervention, she would probably die. I set up the thorocentesis kit as quickly as possible. While I was doing that, I heard Mrs. C say in between gasps for air, "Well, I guess ... I won't ... be seeing ... Christmas." At that point, I did not think that she would even see the next morning.

When I got the needle into her, I began to draw off the fluid. I took off a total of about a half gallon. Within minutes, she started to improve, and the next day she was fine. The fluid did not reaccumulate.

After that night the bond between Mrs. C and me was very strong. Because she had been so close to death and because I had withdrawn the fluid, she attributed her life, rightly or wrongly, to my intervention.

Mrs. C seemed to stabilize over the next few days. Her chest tube was removed, and although some fluid gradually reappeared, she was able to breathe almost normally.

The day she was discharged several doctors and nurses who had taken care of her made a point of going in to say good-bye. In her usual way, she touched us with her way of saying thank you.

After she went home, I did not think about her much until Christmas, when I was on duty all day and night. There I was in the middle of the ten thousand odd things an intern always has to do—and the eleven thousand *extra* things he has to do on a holiday when the staff is shorthanded—when one of the nurses offered me some Christmas cookies from a huge box. They were from Mrs. C. Her note read, "With thanks to all the doctors and nurses who took care of me."

I interpreted her gift to mean that she had lived to see Christmas and spend it with her family. I also understood that this woman possessed the rare ability to reach out to other people. By means of those cookies she was telling us that the most important thing that had remained to her in life had been achieved. And by her gift she was making us a part of it.

As we sat in the nurses' room for a while and munched on those cookies, there was silence instead of the banter we usually exchanged. We were thinking about this woman who had touched us all.

✦ ✦ ✦ ✦ ✦

LITERARY PARALLELS

Had Mrs. C always been such an exceptional person? Perhaps. Probably, in fact. But is is also possible that her cancer had taught her, more deeply and at a younger age than she might have discovered otherwise, the richness of life and of human emotions. Sometimes after a person has been forced to face the prospect of his or her own death, that person grows extraordinarily and discovers—or rediscovers—new meanings in life and in love.

This is what happens toward the end of Solzhenitsyn's monumental novel, *Cancer Ward.* There, thirty-four-year-old Oleg Filimonovich Kostoglotov, a victim of the labor camps, of exile, and of a cancer that will probably kill him soon, emerges not as a victim of life but as a victor in life. This novel is particularly appropriate for our purposes and particularly poignant, for Solzhenitsyn himself was once diagnosed as having cancer, the kind of cancer, in all likelihood, of which his character Kostoglotov is probably dying. In fact, as Solzhenitsyn's assistant wrote to us in a letter dated August 20, 1982, "Although Mr. Solzhenitsyn does not give personal 'interviews' on his personal life, it is safe to assume that the descriptions of Kostoglotov's symptoms (although not of Kostoglotov's biography) corresponds with the author's symptoms."[1]

CANCER WARD

Before one can emerge an emotional victor over cancer, one at first feels the victim. Appropriately, it is the victim who appears in the opening pages of *Cancer Ward*. Although the victim's name here is Pavel Nikolayevich Rusanov, at this point in the novel he is, more than an individual, a symbol of the person who has just learned he has cancer. And that person could be Kostoglotov, or Solzhenitsyn, or Mrs. C, or anyone.

Pavel Nikolayevich Rusanov

"It isn't, it isn't cancer, is it, Doctor? I haven't got cancer?" forty-five-year-old Pavel Nikolayevich Rusanov had asked hopefully in the outpatient clinic just a few days before he had to be admitted to the hospital for lymphoma treatments. And lightly he had touched "the malevolent tumor on the right side of his neck."[2]

Here we sympathize and almost emphathize with Rusanov's terror, denial, and pain. Later in the novel, we shall come to know him for a scoundrel, a member of his factory's "special department" (a euphemism for the KGB), and a man who has risen by denouncing others. But as this new cancer patient enters the hospital, he appears like many middle-class or slightly privileged persons who have just been stricken with the disease they dread most. And we suffer with him.

Only a few weeks before, Rusanov had been self-confident and demanding. As he enters the cancer hospital, however, he appears timid, weak, and dependent.

> [He] remained standing in the waiting room. Timidly he tilted his head slightly to the right and felt the tumor that jutted out between his collarbone and his jaw. He had the impression that in the half hour since he had last looked in the mirror ... [his tumor] seemed to have grown even bigger. Pavel Nikolayevich felt weak and wanted to sit down.[3]

His cancer is changing him, even as it is changing the world in which he must live.

The new patient reacts to the hospital with a combination of disgust, anger, and fear. "Beginning with these slovenly dressing gowns, [Rusanov] ... found everything in the place unpleasant." When he hears a youth screaming, the "screams deafened [him] ... and hurt him so much that it seemed the boy was screaming not with his own pain but with Rusanov's."[4]

His wife and son had accompanied him to the hospital. When they leave, Rusanov feels orphaned and worse: like a prisoner condemned to be beheaded on the scaffold.

> Orphan-like [Rusanov] ... looked back at his family ... and, grasping the banister firmly, started to walk upstairs [to the ward]. His heart was beating violently.... He went up the stairs as people mount—what do they call it?—a sort of platform where men have their heads cut off.[5]

Within hours on the ward, Rusanov "became haunted with fear."[6] Suddenly the reader becomes the patient as Solzhenitsyn slips from the third person ("him") to the second person ("you"). In the passage below, "you" cannot help but identify with the patient, the victim.

> The hard lump of [Rusanov's] ... tumor ... had dragged him in like a fish on a hook and flung him onto this iron bed.... Having once undressed, said goodbye to the family and come up to the ward, you felt the door to all your past life had been slammed behind you, and the life here was so vile that it frightened you more than the actual tumor.[7]

To Rusanov, the hospital is like a prison. But the wall of this metaphorical prison is not really the hospital wall: it is the wall of his tumor, for it is his tumor that imprisons, terrifies, and condemns him to death. In "the space of a few days all [Rusanov's past life] ... had been cut off from him. It was now on the *other* side of his tumor.... However much [his family] ... might worry, fuss or weep, the tumor was growing like a wall behind him, and on his side of it he was alone."[8]

Solzhenitsyn's depictions of Rusanov's isolation, pain, and fear when he first enters the hospital help us understand—and feel—the anguish of the new cancer patient. Because of this, although we do not see Kostoglotov when he first learns he has cancer (nor did we see Solzhenitsyn or Mrs. C at that trying time), we realize that his (and Solzhenitsyn's and Mrs. C's) emotions on first becoming a cancer patient were probably similar, in some ways, to Rusanov's. There is a terrible sense of being trapped by the tumor, of being imprisoned and condemned to death by it, a terrible feeling, therefore, of being a victim.

How can someone who feels himself (or herself) a victim of cancer ever feel—and *be*—a victor in life? We turn to Kostoglotov.

Oleg Filimonovich Kostoglotov

Kostoglotov, age thirty-four, has had a very hard life. For seven years he was a sergeant in World War II. For seven more years he was a prisoner in the labor camps. Now he is exiled "in perpetuity" to Ush-Terek, a remote region of the U.S.S.R. He also has cancer, probably a seminoma.[9]

By the time Kostoglotov arrived at the cancer hospital, he was almost dead. His body was "tormented and twitching with pain" and his "sharp, emaciated face already registered the indifference of death."[10] Here we see and feel—almost viscerally—Kostoglotov as the victim.

After two weeks of radiation therapy in the hospital, however, Oleg Kostoglotov improves dramatically. When he does, he exults in his refound life.

> Oleg had come out for a stroll on the hospital grounds, ... his leg, with each step and stretch, rejoicing at being able to walk firmly, at being the living leg of a man who had not died. ...
>
> He was seized and enveloped by a feeling that life had suddenly returned. ... Though this life promised him nothing

that the people of this great town called good and struggled to acquire: neither apartment, property, social success nor money, there were other joys, sufficient in themselves, which he had not forgotten how to value: the right to move about without waiting for an order; the right to be alone; the right to gaze at stars that were not blinded by prison camp searchlights.[11]

Kostoglotov's joy is all the more profound because he does not prize the superficial things, including possessions and status, that people so often crave. Instead, he values life itself—life free from constant oppression, either by other people or by pain.

But now that Kostoglotov is doing well, he must begin the treatments that Dr. Dontsova (who later discovers that she herself also has cancer) had told him were necessary. "Your tumor is one of the most dangerous kinds of cancer. It is very rapid to develop and acutely malignant, which means secondaries appear very quickly too. Not long ago its mortality rate was reckoned at 95 per cent," Dr. Dontsova had said.[12] She had convinced him that the additional therapy, "a treatment highly recommended for this particular type of cancer by the most up-to-date authorities," would help combat his tumor.[13] Dr. Dontsova had not been completely open with her patient, however, for she had not told him that this up-to-date treatment, hormone therapy, would make him sexually impotent. Only toward the end of his two-month hospitalization does Dr. Dontsova tell him, "speaking softly so that the other patients could not hear ... [,] 'You shouldn't hope to achieve the happiness of a normal family life.' "[14]

During his hospitalization, another female doctor becomes very important to Kostoglotov: Vera Kornilyevna Gangart. "Vega," as Kostoglotov likes to think of her (Vega was a pet name she had once had), is sensitive, lonely, and about Kostoglotov's age. She has never married or made love. An emotional bond develops between them. Shortly before Kostoglotov is discharged, she tells him that on the day he leaves the hospital he may spend the night at her apartment.

It is very early one March morning when Kostoglotov finally steps out of the hospital. He is not cured of his cancer, but he is no longer at death's door. As he walks through the hospital gates, he thinks, "It's just like leaving prison."[15]

Inhaling the spring air, Kostoglotov feels as though he and the entire world were born anew. Time expands. It appears to him to be "the first day of creation."

> [He] looked out at the world—it was new and turning green. . . .
>
> It was the morning of creation. The world had been created anew for one reason only, to be given back to Oleg. "Go out and live!" it seemed to say. . . .
>
> His face radiated happiness. . . .
>
> The first morning of creation—who can act rationally on such a day? Oleg discarded all his plans. Instead, he conceived the mad scheme of going to the Old Town immediately, while it was still early morning, to look at a flowering apricot tree.[16]

With feelings of wonder and excitement, Kostoglotov takes a trolley to the Old Town, walks around, and stops for tea in a teahouse, where he is suddenly exhilarated by the sight of the flowering tree. The vision appears to him no less than a miracle: at once sensuous and pure, fiery and flowering, fragile and yet transcendent. Although the tree is enclosed in a courtyard—imprisoned symbolically—it stretches toward the sky. It might be a symbol of himself.

> [From] the teahouse balcony he saw above the walled courtyard next door something pink and transparent. It looked like a puff dandelion, only it was six meters in diameter. . . .
>
> Could it be the apricot tree?
>
> Oleg had learned a lesson. This was his reward for not hurrying. The lesson was—never rush on without looking about first.

He walked up to the railings and ... gazed and gazed through this pink miracle....

It was like a fire tree decorated with candles in a room in a northern home. The flowering apricot was the only tree in this courtyard enclosed by clay walls and open only to the sky....

Oleg was trying to absorb it all into his eyes. He wanted to remember it for a long time and to tell the Kadmins [fellow exiles in Ush-Terek] about it.[17]

Along with his joy and wonder, two things are striking here. Above all, there is the lesson "never rush on without looking about first." He has learned to appreciate and savor each moment. Then, he wants to share this "miracle" with his friends in Ush-Terek. And so, despite—or perhaps just because of—his past sufferings, he is able to feel for, and to want to communicate with, others who have also suffered. It is a lesson in living and in loving.

After Kostoglotov has tried to absorb—to drink in and incorporate within himself—this miracle, he walks about the town, absorbing in the same way, sensuously and spiritually, the wonders of the world and of life: sights, sounds, smells, tastes, and impressions. Although he may not live to see another spring, he is able to rejoice in this one because it is "a spring he had not reckoned on living to see.... [It] was like a surprise gift, and he was grateful."[18]

The ecstasy does not last. Still, even as his joy wanes and his suffering returns, his new suffering is tempered by the lessons he has just learned. Kostoglotov had wandered about for a long time before finally going to Vera Gangart's apartment. By the time he had gotten there, she had already gone out. (She had told him that she would be in until 4:00 P.M.) He had then left and decided to return later. And he had tried to return, but on his trip back to Vera's, he had had a painful revelation. Riding on the crowded trolley, he had been pressed up close against a young girl and suddenly realized the full—and devastating—effects of his hormone therapy. Through the young girl's worn old clothes he was absorbing her warmth, her softness and her youth. . . .

This sensation—he hadn't felt it, he hadn't had it confirmed for . . . [years]. It was all the more powerful for that, all the stronger.

It was a happiness, and it was a sorrow. There was in the sensation a threshold he could not cross whatever his power of self-suggestion.

They had warned him, hadn't they? The libido remains, the libido but nothing else. . . .

And as he straightened his bent, weakened knees Oleg realized his journey to see Vega would end as a torture and a deceit.

It would mean his demanding more from her than he could ask from himself.[19]

Kostoglotov had gotten off the trolley and had gone to the railroad station where he could board the train that would take him back to Ush-Terek and his exile. It might seem that he is defeated here, that he has lost his joy in, and love of, life. But has he really?

From the railroad station, Kostoglotov sends Vera a note that, by apparently renouncing love, is, in fact, a profound expression of love and kindness. "Darling Vega," it begins. It goes on to explain why he did not return to her apartment that day:

You see, Vega, if I'd found you in, something false and forced might have started between us. . . . What was about to begin between us was something we could never have confessed to anyone. You and I, and between us *this thing*: this sort of gray, decrepit yet ever-growing snake. . . .

You may disagree, but I have a prediction to make: even before you drift into the indifference of old age you will come to bless this day, the day you did not commit yourself to share my life. (I'm not just talking about my exile.) . . .

Now that I'm going away . . . , I can tell you quite frankly: even when we were having the most intellectual conversations . . . , I still wanted all the time, *all the time,* to pick you up and kiss you on the lips. . . .

And now, without your permission, I kiss them.[20]

Thus, although impotent and probably dying of his disease, Kostoglotov is not a victim of cancer but a victor in life. He is able to shun sham and pretense and love life and another person unselfishly. Although he probably does not have much time left to live, during the time remaining he will live life generously, caringly, and feelingly. What more can any of us do during the time—however long or short—we have left?

SOME LESSONS FROM THE CANCER WARD

In a sense, Rusanov, Kostoglotov, and Mrs. C are all victims. We see and feel their suffering. But, we come to appreciate, a victim is not necessarily someone who is dying.

Throughout his novel, Solzhenitsyn uses the prison metaphor to describe the cancer ward and, beyond it, life itself. Frequently, the patient is depicted as a victim, a prisoner of cancer. Cut off from ordinary life, imprisoned in a hospital, walled in by his tumor, the patient feels condemned to death. In *Cancer Ward,* however, Solzhenitsyn uses his metaphor to describe not only the experience of facing cancer but also the experience of facing life, for facing life also implies, eventually, facing death. "We die daily; . . . while we are growing, our life decreases; every moment that passes takes away part of it; . . . nay, we divide with death the very instant that we live."[21] A victim, therefore, is not merely someone who is going to die. We are all going to die. A victim is someone who does not know how to live. And knowing how to live, we intuit from Kostoglotov and Mrs. C, means knowing how to love life and other people.

A person may be a victor, then, even though he or she may be dying of cancer. "You do not die of being sick, you die of being alive. Death kills you well enough without the help of illness."[22] Even though we are all dying, we need not consider ourselves victims, for the cancer ward has illustrated how a person who has learned to savor life and to care for others can be a victor in life and in the lives of those he or she touches, as long as he or she lives and afterward.

9

"AM I IN HEAVEN NOW?"

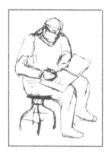

✦ ✦ ✦ ✦ ✦

CASE HISTORY

An intern usually works on a team with two other interns, and the team as a whole is responsible for a certain service or ward. Every third day and night, one intern is on call. During those twenty-four hours he works up any new patient who comes in. An intern knows his own patients best, of course, but he also gets to know some of his fellow interns' patients quite well because on rounds each day the entire team sees everyone's patients and at night, when on call, he takes care of all patients on the service.

Sometimes one patient becomes the team's favorite, and the interns and that patient develop a very warm relationship. On morning rounds, all the doctors look forward to going into that patient's room. It is almost like visiting a friend. That is what happened when I was an intern on the C.C.U. Our favorite patient there was Mr. L, an eighty-four-year-old retired carpenter. He had been admitted for a myocardial infarction by my fellow intern, Dr. Miller.

Why did we all like Mr. L so much? I think it was because he was always very friendly and always had a kind word for everyone. In addition, he had a delightful sense of humor, and we enjoyed exchanging quips and gibes with him.

As the days of Mr. L's hospitalization went by, we learned that he had lived a full, rich life. We also saw that he did not seem to regret or to be at all bitter that he was now coming to the end of it. He did not even seem to be bothered by the fear that possesses most patients in the C.C.U.—the fear they might die at any moment. In sum, Mr. L was one of those rare elderly people who seem to recognize how fortunate they have been. He had not been sick before and was not in pain now. He seemed to be enjoying every minute of life, even now.

Later, I realized that a patient like Mr. L—someone who does not appear to fear his own death—probably puts the medical staff more at ease because his relaxed state of mind takes some of the burden off the doctors and removes some of the tenseness and fear from the relationship. After all, it is never easy when a patient thinks of you—the physician—as the sole barrier standing between himself and the Angel of Death.

Of course, there were good reasons—selfish ones—that we enjoyed going to see Mr. L. Not the least of these was that on rounds in the C.C.U. interns take care of a lot of very sick people who are obviously extremely miserable. Just seeing Mr. L, therefore, with his cheerful nature, relaxed outlook, and spry sense of humor was a relief, even a delight.

By his fourth day in the C.C.U., Mr. L was doing pretty well, and we were thinking about transferring him to the regular medical floor. We had discussed that possibility at morning rounds. Around noon that day, I looked for Dr. Miller because I wanted to eat lunch with him. After searching everywhere, I finally found him in Mr. L's room.

A very strange scene greeted me. In the middle of the room was Mr. L, half-reclining, half-rising on his pillow. Next to him, near the head of the bed, stood Dr. Miller surrounded by several nurses who were hovering about like seraphim. As I entered the room, Mr. L was smiling and thanking everybody for being so kind and for taking such good care of him. After finishing, he turned to each person and said good-bye individually. When he noticed me, he also thanked me and said good-bye.

"Where do you think you are going, Mr. L?" I asked.

"I'll be dying shortly," he answered.

Dr. Miller whispered to me that he had just checked Mr. L over and had found nothing wrong. His vital signs were completely stable, and he was not complaining of any pain or of anything at all. In fact, he had *no* complaints. Yet for some reason, he thought he was going to die.

Naturally, we all reassured him that nothing was wrong.

"The only place you'll be going, Mr. L," Dr. Miller said, "is to the regular medical floor, and that's because you've been doing so well."

Mr. L just smiled and continued to thank us and say good-bye.

After several minutes of convincing ourselves that nothing was amiss, Miller and I left for the cafeteria. About ten minutes later, there was an emergency call from the C.C.U. to the cafeteria. Since Miller and I were on the same team and were eating together, we answered the *Stat* call together.

"Mr. L has become hypotensive and is unconscious," the voice on the telephone said. Hypotension itself is always a significant warning sign that a patient in the C.C.U. may be in terrible difficulty.

We rushed back to the unit. There, we went through the usual procedures to maintain a patient's blood pressure, and after a while, Mr. L. began to stabilize. Eventually, he also regained consciousness. When he woke up, he looked right up at Dr. Miller and asked, with a look of wonder on his face, "Oh, am I in heaven now?"

"If you can see Dr. Miller, you can't *possibly* be in heaven," I answered.

Perhaps that humor was inappropriate, but we had always joked with Mr. L, and the words just came out. Anyway, all the medical staff in the room (including Miller, three or four nurses, and Dr. Smith, the resident on our service) smiled.

Mr. L did not react at all. He merely said good-bye to everyone again, closed his eyes, and died.

We tried to resuscitate him but were unsuccessful.

Later, when Miller and I left the room, we were completely thunderstruck. How had Mr. L. known, when we hadn't known anything at all? How had he had that presentiment?

> Presentiment—is that long shadow—on the Lawn—
> Indicative that Suns go down—
>
> The Notice to the startled Grass
> That Darkness—is about to pass—[1]

I have often thought about that case. Now, years later, I see in Mr. L's dying a symbol of how he had lived: even in dying, he had shown his delight in, and consideration for, life. In fact, his dying was the nicest, most easeful death I have ever seen, at once earthbound and elevating. What was the secret of his serenity in dying?

+ + + + +

LITERARY PARALLELS

It might appear to be easy to find cases in literature where dying appears both earthbound and elevating, but it is not. For we wish to shun what is melodramatic or didactic, moralizing or sermonizing, too consciously artistic or intellectualistic. What we wanted to find was something as unadorned and uplifting as Mr. L's last days: a dying that is a simple, yet richly human reflection of living.

We found examples in works by two very different writers: Ivan Turgenev (1818–1883), the Russian novelist and storywriter who lived for long stretches of time in Paris and Baden-Baden, and Emily Dickenson (1830–1886), the American poet who sequestered herself for much of her adult life in her father's house in Amherst, Massachusetts.

IVAN TURGENEV

In "Death," one of the stories in Turgenev's *A Sportsman's Sketches,* the sportsman-narrator relates several cases in which people faced death calmly or showed, at the approach of death, a tremendous concern for life and the living.

The first case focuses on apparently worldly, yet finely human, details. The narrator is visiting his friend, the surgeon Kapiton. A peasant, Vassily Dmitritch, arrives. After Kapiton has examined the peasant, he tells him that his condition is serious and he ought to stay in the hospital. But the wary surgeon also warns Vassily Dmitritch that he "can't answer for anything."

> "So bad as that?" muttered the astounded peasant. . . . [Vassily Dmitritch] pondered and pondered, his eyes fixed on the floor, then he . . . picked up his cap. "Where you are off to, Vassily Dmitritch?" "Where? why home to be sure, if it's so bad. I must put things to right, if it's like that." "But you'll do yourself harm, Vassily Dmitritch; you will, really. . . ." "No, . . . Kapiton . . . , if I must die, I'll die at home." . . . The peasant . . . gave Kapiton half-a-rouble, went out of the room, and took his seat in the cart. "Well, good-bye, Kapiton . . . , don't remember evil against me, and remember my orphans, if anything. . . ." Three days later he was dead.[2]

What is striking here is the way in which Vassily Dmitritch confronts the news of his impending death. Exhibiting neither fear nor anger, he displays a self-possession and an attention to material concerns that are at once practical and spiritual. He wants to return home to set his affairs "to right," and instead of grieving for himself, he thinks about his children, who will be orphans. His concern for the material is not selfish, therefore, but selfless. In addition, Vassily Dmitritch seems to accept death as a natural part of life, as something that is inevitable and therefore not really unexpected, whenever it comes. Perhaps this helps explain why he is able to face the news of his approaching death with calmness, self-control, and an overriding concern for others.

The narrator relates another quietly moving acceptance of death. In this case, religion and practical concerns for life mingle simply and sublimely.

> I was present at an old lady's death-bed; the priest had begun reading the prayers for the dying over her, but, suddenly no-

ticing that the patient seemed to be actually dying, he made haste to give her the cross to kiss. The lady turned away with an air of displeasure. "You're in too great a hurry, father," she said, in a voice almost inarticulate; "in too great a hurry." . . . She kissed the cross, put her hand under her pillow and expired. Under the pillow was a silver rouble; she had meant to pay the priest for the service at her own death.[3]

The lady's calmness in dying forms a wonderful contrast to the priest's evident anxiety, his rushing to give her the cross. Further, her kissing the cross and reaching immediately after for the silver rouble to pay the priest reveal a self-possessed calmness at once worldly and spiritual.

It is possible, of course, that these deaths are romanticized, to some degree, by the sportsman-narrator; however, both dying people display an undeniable earthiness and materiality. Each exhibits a practical attention to physical and human concerns, including possessions, feelings, and other people. Perhaps it is their devotion to life and to other people that enable Vassily Dmitritch and the old Russian lady to face death in ways that are so calm and practical—and also sublime.

But what if a person who is devoted to life and the human existence is afraid of dying? Can that person arrive at a sense of calmness in the face of death? Emily Dickinson gives us some answers to these questions, for in some of her poems she tries out, as it were, the experience of dying. In addition, she probes the problem of death itself.

EMILY DICKINSON

Despite her secretive life, Emily Dickinson establishes in her poetry an extraordinary intimacy with her reader. She does this, partly, by her constant probings of human joys, emotions, and problems. These probings were related to her own life.

Reared in the Puritan tradition that taught man to see "life as a preparation,"[4] Emily Dickinson often wrote about

God, immortality, and eternity; she sought to apprehend life—and death—in terms of the infinite. But she also rejected aspects of Puritanism. For example, for the most part, she renounced religious formalism; ceased going to church altogether by the time she was thirty; and instead of disparaging life on earth, sang its praises lyrically and joyfully. One of the most striking things about her poetry is her intense, even passionate, love of life and life's sensations. We see and feel that love, for instance, in the following poem, in which the narrator revels sensuously and ecstatically in her indulgence in nature and in life:

> I taste a liquor never brewed—
> From Tankards scooped in Pearl—
> Not all the Vats upon the Rhine
> Yield such an Alcohol!
>
> Inebriate of Air—am I—
> And Debauchee of Dew—
> Reeling—thro endless summer days—
> From inns of Molten Blue— . . . [5]

Although one senses throughout Dickinson's poetry her impassioned love of life, one senses just as strongly her constant concern with death. She portrayed death essentially in two ways: as an existential phenomenon, the experience of dying itself, and as the central religious mystery, the emblem of the resurrection.

In several poems (including "I felt a Funeral, in my Brain . . . ," "I heard a Fly buzz—when I died—," and "The Sun kept setting—setting—still . . . "), the poet portrays herself undergoing the physical, emotional, and cognitive sensations of dying. It is almost as though she were trying to feel, and in that way come to terms with, the act of dying before the fact itself.

The most fear-filled of these poems is "I felt a Funeral, in my Brain . . . ":

> I felt a Funeral, in my Brain,
> And Mourners to and fro

Kept treading—treading—till it seemed
That Sense was breaking through—

And when they all were seated,
A Service, like a Drum—
Kept beating—beating—till I thought
My Mind was going numb—

And then I heard them lift a Box
And creak across my Soul
With those same Boots of Lead, again,
Then Space—began to toll,

As all the Heavens were a Bell,
And Being, but an Ear,
And I, and Silence, some strange Race
Wrecked, solitary, here—

And then a Plank in Reason, broke,
And I dropped down, and down—
And hit a World, at every plunge,
And Finished knowing—then—[6]

The first four stanzas convey through sounds, images, and repetitions the poet's terror. With hallucinatory intensity, she feels a funeral "treading—treading" in her skull, invading her mind and her senses. Like the pounding of her heart, a mournful service keeps "beating—beating" until she thinks she is losing her mind. Her terror mounts in stanzas three and four as the coffin is lifted and sounds and silence clash in her solitary soul. Suddenly, however, there is a kind of relief, in the form of a release. As the narrator's reason collapses in the last stanza, and she feels herself plunging "down, and down," she loses consciousness. Because of that loss, she is freed from her fear: she "finished knowing—then—." What this poem dramatizes is that even if the experience of dying may be initially terrifying, it is ultimately easeful. For the dying person loses consciousness and, therefore, fear.

In "The Sun kept setting—setting—still . . . ," Dickinson depicts, through repetitions and descriptions of nature and herself, her slipping away from life and from her bodily sensations. We sense around her and in her a feeling of falling, failing, and loss. But in this poem, Dickinson does not seem to fear dying. In fact, in the last two lines, she realizes that she is dying, "but," she says, she is "not afraid to know."

> The Sun kept setting—setting—still
> No Hue of Afternoon—
> Upon the Village I perceived—
> From House to House 'twas Noon—
>
> The Dusk kept dropping—dropping—still
> No Dew upon the Grass—
> But only on my Forehead stopped—
> And wandered in my Face—
>
> My Feet kept drowsing—drowsing—still
> My fingers were awake—
> Yet why so little sound—Myself
> Unto my Seeming—make?
>
> How well I knew the Light before—
> I could see it now—
> 'Tis Dying—I am doing—but
> I'm not afraid to know—[7]

In these poems Dickinson faced and, in a sense, overcame her fear of dying in existential terms. In some other poems she pondered the problem in religious terms, and, what is even more fascinating, she explored death, dying, and afterlife in terms of life itself.

To the believer, of course, the ultimate consolations for physical death are immortality and eternity. Although we can see these beliefs in many of Dickinson's poems, we wish to focus on how the poet viewed the relationship between earth and her vision of heaven. This is evident in "I never saw a Moor—," a poem in which Dickinson says she felt certain she would find heaven, as if the trail had been clearly marked for her.

> I never saw a Moor—
> I never saw the Sea—

> Yet know I how the Heather looks
> And what a Billow be.
>
> I never spoke with God
> Nor visited in Heaven—
> Yet certain am I of the spot
> As if the Checks were given—[8]

What is fascinating here is the parallel Dickinson draws between nature and heaven, that is, she knows about heaven in the same way she knows about life on earth.

This parallel points out something very important about Emily Dickinson: her ideas about God and heaven are intimately related to her ideas about life and living. Indeed, she maintained, heaven was to be sought—and found—in life "below" on earth.

> Who has not found the Heaven—below—
> Will fail of it above—
> For Angels rent the House next ours,
> Wherever we remove—[9]

It is not surprising, then, that Dickinson often overcame her anxieties about death and dying by drawing strength from her love of life, living, and other people. We see this, for example, in "Of Death I try to think like this—," a poem in which the poet conquers her fear of death by thinking about it in terms of what she understands and loves: life. In the first stanza, she compares death to a brook that invites just because it inspires fear, but that very fear, she adds, is spiced with sweetness. She concludes this stanza by saying that the brook that lures us to danger is there only to welcome and entice us to a better place: the heavenly realm where the "Flower Hesperian" grows. In the second stanza, the narrator draws strength by recalling how when she was a timid child her bolder playmates would brave all, including possible drowning, to leap across a brook that seemed like a sea to her and grasp an alluring flower. Thus, she implies, reaching out toward death would be no more frightening than what her playmates used to do: clutch that "flower beyond."

> Of Death I try to think like this—
> The Well in which they lay us
> Is but the Likeness of the Brook
> That menaced not to slay us,
> But to invite by that Dismay
> Which is the Zest of sweetness
> To the same Flower Hesperian,
> Decoying but to greet us—
>
> I do remember when a Child
> With bolder Playmates straying
> To where a Brook that seemed a Sea
> Withheld us by its roaring
> From just a Purple Flower beyond
> Until constrained to clutch it
> If Doom itself were the result,
> The boldest leaped, and clutched it—[10]

Several things helped Dickinson to overcome her anxieties about death and dying. In existential terms, she found solace in realizing that because dying brings the loss of both feeling and consciousness, it also brings the loss of fear. In religious terms, she found strength not only in her beliefs in God, heaven, and eternity but also, and above all, perhaps, in her love of life and of other people. For her, the heaven "above" was inseparable from the "Heaven—below." Death, therefore, was a natural part of life and, by extension, heaven, a natural part of earth.

OF DEATH AND LIFE

We think back to Mr. L and then to Turgenev's characters and Dickinson's poems. It is possible that they all were calm or could become calm when facing or thinking about death just because they all had cared so much about life, living, and other people. Maybe that is the reason their deaths or thoughts about death could be at once earthbound and elevating. Perhaps nothing illustrates this idea better than Dickinson's poem that celebrates such an experience. Although the lyric below is ultimately concerned with death and getting to heaven, it is devoted, timelessly, to life.

> Some keep the Sabbath going to Church—
> I keep it, staying at Home—
> With a Bobolink for a Chorister—
> And an Orchard, for a Dome—
>
> Some keep the Sabbath in Surplice—
> I just wear my Wings—
> And instead of tolling the Bell, for Church,
> Our little Sexton—sings.
>
> God preaches, a noted Clergyman—
> And the sermon is never long,
> So instead of getting to Heaven at last—
> I'm going, all along.[11]

10

THE SURVIVOR

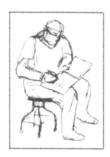

✛ ✛ ✛ ✛ ✛

CASE HISTORY

I was a resident in radiation therapy at a large university teaching hospital when Mr. D, age sixty, became my patient for a fairly advanced bladder cancer. His urologist had recommended surgery, but Mr. D had refused. Because his tumor was quite advanced, his prognosis was not very good no matter what we did.

Mr. D came in with his wife. During the usual history taking and physical examination it struck me that he was a very peculiar person. I had the impression that he wanted to say more than he was actually saying. Finally, when we started talking about why he had refused surgery, Mr. D said that to explain he had to tell me something about his life. He realized, he said, that we might think his decision strange, and he wanted me to understand.

During World War II, around the time of the attack on Pearl Harbor, Mr. D had been a combat soldier in the Philippines. He had surrendered with the American troops on Bataan Peninsula in April 1942, had been on the Bataan Death March, where he had seen thousands of men die, and had remained a prisoner of the

Japanese for three-and-a-half years, until the end of the war. He said he could not really talk about what he had seen or experienced, but he knew he had never been the same since then. He admitted that he was an impossible person to live with and that he had made life very difficult for his wife and children. Over and over, he said he knew he was strange and his behavior was strange, but what had happened on Bataan was so horrible that nobody could understand what he had been through. Because of that he could not accept surgery. He could not stand any more pain or suffering.

His wife was very supportive. It was obvious that she had gone through a lot with him over the years.

During his treatments, which lasted about seven weeks, I saw Mr. D about once a week. Each time he said the same thing; he apologized for his behavior so often it seemed as though he were apologizing for being alive. Always, he referred to Bataan but never elaborated. He just repeated that awful things had happened.

After his treatments, Mr. D did well for about six months until he again began to experience bleeding from the bladder. We repeated some tests. They showed that his cancer had recurred and was growing rapidly. He quickly deteriorated. What was worse, he began to have constant intractable pain. We put him in the hospital to give him as much pain medication as possible. His tumor kept spreading. It struck me that, after having lived through the horrors of Bataan and having suffered a terrible life as a result, Mr. D was now dying a horrible, painful death. Despite all the advances of medical science, there was very little we could do to help besides give him pain medication, and even that was not very effective.

I remember going to see Mr. D when he was quite close to death. He was in a lot of pain, and I felt as though he were projecting all his pain and suffering onto me, as though he were blaming me for how miserable he was and for everything that was happening. As I talked with him, I had the impression that during the thirty-five or so years since Bataan, this man had blamed himself for having survived or at least had felt guilty about it. Now, because I was surviving him, he seemed to wish to transfer all that anger and guilt onto me. He made me feel terrible.

The day before he died, Mr. D looked right at me and said, "Oh, I had a lot of confidence in you, and you really let me down."

That was the last thing he ever said to me.

Then and later, I tried to wipe his words and his look from my mind, but now and then, like avenging furies, they come back to gnaw at me. Because this man had lived through terrible events, he viewed life differently from most people. His survivor's outlook had had a profound impact not only on his behavior but also on his relationship to life.

Yet why was I, a doctor, not a former prisoner of war, so disturbed by this survivor?

✛ ✛ ✛ ✛ ✛

BATAAN

Although Mr. D could not translate into words the horrors of his past, some other survivors of Bataan did. Through their words we may begin to get a picture of, and a feeling for, what Mr. D saw and survived. The narrative below is composed of historical facts combined with the recollections of numerous survivors of the Bataan Death March.

On April 9, 1942, about 10,000 American troops surrendered to the Japanese on Bataan Peninsula in the Philippines. After three-and-one-half years of imprisonment, only about 4,000 survived. What had happened during the interval?

After the surrender, the Japanese made the prisoners march some sixty miles to a rail line that would take them to Camp O'Donnell. This forced march of approximately 72,000 men—10,000 Americans plus some 62,000 Filipinos who had also surrendered on Bataan—is known to history as the Death March. On it, thousands died: approximately 600 to 700 Americans and between 5,000 and 10,000 Filipinos.[1]

It was beastly hot on the Death March, but the Japanese allowed the prisoners almost no food or water. Parched, famished, and exhausted, many of the prisoners were—or became—very sick. They were made to sit or stand in the tropical sun for hours. At times, they were forced to run. Any prisoner who fell behind was bayoneted. Death was everywhere. It "got so bad . . . that you never got away from the stench of death."²

At night, the prisoners were herded into a "bullpen. . . . There was a lot of dust, dirt, filth on the ground. Everybody had dysentery. There were no toilets. It was absolutely horrible. . . . [P]eople . . . were screaming and going nuts. . . . It was like being in a cage with animals."³

When the prisoners arrived at Camp O'Donnell, things got even worse. "In O'Donnell our boys were dying forty, fifty, sixty a day. We couldn't bury them fast enough."⁴ "I buried so many of my friends. . . . The shock of it was hell."⁵

Later, many of the Americans were sent to Cabanatuan, another POW camp. Illnesses were rampant: diphtheria, malaria, dysentery, beriberi, and dry beriberi. The survivors of the Death March were "like walking zombies. Skeletons walking towards you with skin hanging on the bones. . . . Heads looked like skulls."⁶

To survive one often had to be merciless. Sometimes Americans stole from each other. "There wasn't much stealing because there wasn't much available. But there was a certain amount. I'm sure many a man who swiped something carries the guilt with him today."⁷

As the war progressed, the Japanese began to fear that the Americans would recapture the Philippines, and they shipped their American prisoners to Japan. The boats on which they were sent became known as the Hell Ships. How can one describe these ships?

How do I describe a packed, hot, filthy, stinking ship's hold that turned slowly into a mad house? . . . Most of the guys won't or can't talk about them. . . . They put 500 of us in one hold and 500 in the other. . . . Tropical sun on a steel deck. Body heat from 500 men packed together. All around men began passing out. . . . It must have been 120 or 125 degrees in that hold. The Jap's favorite trick was to cut off our water.... [People went crazy.] The next guy that went screaming by ... [was] caught and killed [by his fellow prisoners.] ... Several others were also killed.[8]

On another Hell Ship, men "went mad. Some drank urine. Some turned vampire."[9] "One person near me cut another person's throat and was holding his canteen so he could catch the blood."[10]

When their Hell Ships reached Japan, the Americans had to perform hard labor in the coal mines, steel mills, and elsewhere. "Being beaten was something you understood would happen to you daily. You were either going to get slapped or you were going to get beaten on the head with a sledgehammer handle."[11]

When the war finally ended, some new heartaches began for the former POWs. Long after their liberation, many survivors had trouble relating to people or were haunted by nightmares and fears.

I couldn't talk to people. I couldn't even talk to my parents.... I couldn't get along with anybody.[12]

It wasn't anger as much as it was fear.... There were no psychiatrists waiting for us.... I was so goddamn nervous.... I couldn't sleep.[13]

I spent a year in the Army hospital.... [The doctors said I was fine.] ... I felt rotten all the time.... I used to sleep walk at night and had those hallucinations.... In the hallucinations I would meet dead men walking down the street.... [I]t kept happening, in broad daylight.[14]

Some of the survivors married and made life a hell for their families.

I got married in March of '46. Then I neglected my wife miserably.... I've asked my wife many times since those days how come she kept on.... No other woman would have stayed with me.[15]

Even after thirty or more years, some of the nightmares of their captivity, both physical and mental, remained.

I still get captured about once every month. Actually, it's harder on my wife. I never wake up, but she does. She doesn't know how to cope with this nightmare. . . . I'd venture to guess that there's something wrong with all of us, each and every one of us who survived. A human mind can't go through what we went through without something being wrong. . . . I've got sense enough to know that I'm not all I ought to be.[16]

Had Mr. D been able to articulate his experiences and emotions, these are some of the things he might have said, some of the death encounters he might have described. Although the specifics of Bataan are unique to the survivors of Bataan, these people exhibit certain traits that are often found in other survivors. Among them are frequent references to death, suffering, fear, pain, anxiety, guilt, and the unforgettable memory of a death-marked past. Psychiatry and literature offer further insights into the survivor's world.

THE SURVIVOR AND THE DEATH IMPRINT

According to Robert Jay Lifton, the psychiatrist noted for his studies of the survivors of Hiroshima and for what he calls "the general psychology of the survivor": "We may define the survivor as one who has come into contact with death in some bodily or psychic fashion and has remained alive. . . . The key to the survivor experience . . . is the imprint of death."[17] Typical among the survivor's traits, Lifton finds, are the death imprint, death anxiety, death guilt, a life of grief, and psychic numbing. Very briefly, these traits may be characterized as follows:

1. The death imprint, which is "indelible," results from the survivor's "extraordinary immersion in death."[18]
2. Death anxiety is the result of the survivor feeling a "sense of heightened vulnerability" to the world around him and, above all, to his own death.[19]

3. Death guilt describes the survivor's struggle with guilt for having survived while others died or for having survived, perhaps, at another person's expense. It is the guilt "over what one has done to, or not done for, the dying while oneself surviving."[20] In addition, death guilt captures how the survivor feels guilty about feeling *glad* that he is alive: he knows "the tainted joy of having survived amid others' deaths."[21] Lifton calls this combination of guilt and gladness the survivor's "guilt over survival priority," that is, the survivor feels guilty—but also glad—that he made survival his first priority.[22]

4. The survivor's "life of grief" characterizes how the survivor mourns not only for the dead who were close to him but also for the anonymous dead and for "a way of life that has been 'killed.'" In sum, he mourns for his former self, for what he was prior to the intrusion of death and death conflicts.[23] Surviving, therefore, is a kind of terrible rite de passage during which one self dies symbolically and a new self—a sadder self forever imprinted with the image of death—is born. For these reasons, surviving always involves a terrible sense of loss and grief.

5. Psychic numbing, which is "the cessation of feeling," comes to "characterize the entire life style of the survivor," according to Lifton.[24] Psychic numbing describes the cessation of feeling in its chronic form, psychic closing off in its acute form. These psychic processes are defense mechanisms through which a person shuts himself off from death itself: "the unconscious message is, 'If I feel nothing, then death is not taking place.'"[25] Still, although psychic closing off and psychic numbing are protective mechanisms, they are also, in a way, destructive processes because they themselves are a "form of symbolic death."[26] After all, if a person is numbed, he not only *feels less* but he also feels *less alive.*

With the Bataan experiences and Lifton's insights in mind, it is possible to enter deeper into the world of the survivor, this time through literature. Because literature not only reflects life, and reflects upon life, but also heightens and deepens our perceptions of life, we feel that literature, more than any other medium, can help us understand the death-imprinted world of the survivor. We therefore enter the universe of Elie Wiesel, survivor of the Holocaust.

ELIE WIESEL

Elie Wiesel was born in Sighet, Transylvania. When in his teens, he was deported with his family and the other Jews of his community to Auschwitz and then to Buchenwald. His father, mother, and younger sister died in the concentration camps.

· *Night* is the tale of his life—or rather death-life—in those camps. His first night in Auschwitz indelibly stamped him with the imprint of death that would cloud the rest of his life.

> Never shall I forget that night, the first night in camp, which has turned my life into one long night, seven times cursed and seven times sealed. Never shall I forget that smoke. Never shall I forget the little faces of the children, whose bodies I saw turned into wreaths of smoke beneath a silent blue sky. . . . Never.[27]

For months, Wiesel and his father survived together in the camps, though just barely. The adolescent saw thousands die, and he witnessed countless people fight or harm each other in their struggles to survive. When forced by the Nazis to run for miles through snow and freezing rain, he saw a son, who was stronger than his father, purposely outrun his father so that he would not be held back by the old man and, like the old man, killed. When packed together, starved, dehydrated, and freezing in an uncovered cattle wagon in the middle of winter, he saw a son kill his own father to steal from him a scrap of bread. Images of death never leave his eyes.

Searingly, Wiesel describes his ambivalent feelings about his own father. When his father was dying, he realized that he—like the boy who had purposely outrun his old father—would also feel relieved to be rid of him because his father was consuming some of his energy, which he himself desperately needed to try to survive. We sense here not only Wiesel's feelings of guilt but also his intense and smoldering anger at the inhuman world around him, at his father for being weak, and, perhaps most of all and everlastingly, at himself. They had arrived at Buchenwald, and on their first night there Wiesel had been separated from his father. The next day, he says,

> I had followed the crowd without troubling about him. I had known that he was ... on the brink of death, and yet I had abandoned him.
>
> I went to look for him.
>
> But at the same moment this thought came into my mind. "Don't let me find him! If only I could get rid of this dead weight, so that I could use all my strength to struggle for my own survival, and only worry about myself." Immediately I felt ashamed of myself, ashamed forever.[28]

Wiesel did find his father, and some days later his father died. Wiesel explains how he then felt a horrible feeling of liberation. The last word he had heard his father utter was his own name: "Eliezer." A Nazi official had been beating his father, and the dying man had called out for his son. But Elie had not gone to help his father because his own "body was afraid of also receiving a blow."[29] When he awoke at dawn the next day, his father's body was gone. Numbed as he was, the son could not weep about his father's death— or about anything—although he did feel some vestigial twinges of guilt.

I did not weep, and it pained me that I could not weep. But I had no more tears. And, in the depths of my being, in the recesses of my weakened conscience, could I have searched it, I might perhaps have found something like—free at last!

After his liberation, Wiesel saw himself as still bound—forever bound—to death. He had not looked at himself in a mirror since he and his family had been routed from their homes in Sighet. When he did look for the first time, what he saw when he gazed at himself in the mirror—and what he would continue to see ever after—was the face of a corpse: "from the depths of the mirror, a corpse gazed back at me. The look in his eyes, as they stared into mine, has never left me."[30]

Several of Wiesel's fictions continue the survivor's story, while delving into different aspect of the survivor's world. His novel *The Accident* is particularly rich. In this first-person tale, the narrator, like Wiesel, is a survivor of the concentration camps. A beautiful woman named Kathleen loves him, but he is unable to really love her or anyone because his past seems more real to him than the present. When he is run over by a taxi and almost killed, his accident (or was it a suicide attempt?) is a mere trifle to him in comparison to the death-life he came to know in the camps. Forever haunted by his death-imprinted past, he wants to go "where I can think about myself without anguish, without contempt: where the wine . . . is pure and not mixed with the spit of corpses; where the dead live in cemeteries and not in the hearts and memories of men."[31]

Survivors, he says, are different from other people.

[They are the] living-dead. You must look at them carefully. Their appearance is deceptive. . . . They look like the others. They eat, they laugh, they love. . . . Like the others. But it isn't true. . . . Anyone who has seen what they have seen cannot be like the others. . . . You have to watch them carefully when they pass by an innocent-looking smokestack, or when they lift a piece of bread to their mouths. Something in them shudders and makes you turn your eyes away. These people have been amputated; they haven't lost their legs or eyes but their will and their taste for life. The things they have seen will come to the surface again sooner or later. And then the world will be frightened and won't dare look these spiritual cripples in the eye.[32]

The survivor is, according to Wiesel, a numbed person, a wounded person, an amputee, a "spiritual cripple." Because of his death-imprinted past, he is deprived of the capacity for joy, hope, or ecstasy. (We think here of Mr. D.)

In the extreme, the survivor's bondage to his death-marked past leads to madness, Wiesel says. For not only can the survivor *not* forget: he also *never wants to forget.*

With us—those who have known the time of death— ... [things are] different. There, we said we would never forget. It still holds true. We cannot forget. The images are there in front of our eyes. ... I think if I were able to forget I would hate myself. Our stay there planted time bombs within us. From time to time one of them explodes. And then we are nothing but suffering, shame, and guilt. We feel ashamed and guilty to be alive, to eat as much bread as we want, to wear good, warm socks in the winter. One of these bombs ... will undoubtedly bring about madness. It's inevitable.[33]

"We feel ashamed and guilty to be alive." Wiesel's words name, in their starkness, anguish, and honesty, some of the survivor's continuing torments and anxieties. If Mr. D had been able to verbalize his feelings, he too might have voiced some of these same searing sentiments.

We return to the question: Why did Mr. D's doctor remain haunted by his death-imprinted patient? Might a doctor also, in a way, be imprinted with death? In other words, might a doctor be a kind of survivor?

"The key to the survivor experience ... is the imprint of death," wrote Lifton. That indelible imprint is the result of the survivor's extraordinary immersion in death. What does a physician experience that could resemble such an immersion and leave such an imprint?

We immediately think of some of the physican's earliest experiences during his training, his months spent with the cadavers of anatomy class, those all too palpable—and real—images of the death that is man's inevitable fate. We think, too, of the doctor's further training and encounters, his days and nights on the hospital wards where he comes to know, intimately, the rhythms, sights, sounds, and scents of suffering, pain, disease, dying, and death. In a way, then, we begin to feel that because of the doctor's exposure to and, in a sense, immersion in death (hands and mind plunged into the cavity of the cadaver), the doctor may be a kinsman of the survivor or even a kind of survivor himself. We find signs of that kinship in the words of some doctor-writers.

DOCTORS AND SURVIVORS

Oliver St. John Gogarty (1878–1957), who roomed with James Joyce for two years and became the model for Buck Mulligan in *Ulysses*, was a poet, novelist, essayist, Irish senator, and practicing physician. Into his witty novel about medical school life, *Tumbling in the Hay*, he inserts a poignant vision of the doctor as a death-imprinted survivor. In the passage below, a professor of medicine warns his students that because of their experiences as physicians, their lives will be forever changed. Different from the layperson, they will always see in life the relentless pull of the grave. More, they will recognize that their struggles against disease and death can never really be victorious because, eventually, death always wins. He tells his students:

> Turn back now if you are not prepared and resigned to devote your lives to the contemplation of pain, suffering and squalor. . . . Your outlook on life will have none of the deception that is the unconscious support of the layman: to you all life

will appear in transit. . . . You will see . . . the pull of the grave
that never lets up for one moment, draw down the cheeks and
the corners of the mouth and bend the back until you behold
beauty abashed and life itself caricatured in the spectacle of
the living looking down on the sod as if to find a grave. . . .
You can never retreat from the world, which is for you a bat-
tlefield on which you must engage in a relentless and un-
ceasing war from which you know that you can never emerge
victorious.[34]

William Carlos Williams also exhibits signs of the death
imprint. When the doctor-author thinks about his "cases / At
the hospital" in his poem "The Visit," he calls himself "a
spade-worker."[35] His story "Danse Pseudomacabre" is clearly
marked by death, for the title evokes and appears to mock
the medieval tableaux that were called danse macabre, the
dance of death or the dance of the dead (see chap. 2,
above). In the medieval danse macabre, a figure of death
was depicted with its mortal victims. The aim of the art and
the accompanying verses was to make people fear death
and think about their eternal salvation. In Williams's "Danse
Pseudomacabre," the doctor is awakened by the telephone
in the middle of the night. As he rouses himself, he exhibits
several traits often associated with survivors—he appears
numbed, anxious, grief stricken, and filled with thoughts of
death. "I have awakened . . . unsurprised, almost uninter-
ested, but with an overwhelming sense of death pressing my
chest together as if I had come reluctant from the grave to
which a distorted homesickness continued to drag me, a
sense as of the end of everything."[36] Seeing his wife sleeping
beside him, he contemplates sadly and fearfully her inevitable death and his own. "Christ! Christ! how can I ever bear
to be separated from this my boon companion, to be annihilated, to have her annihilated? How can a man live in
the face of this daily uncertainty? How can a man not go
mad with grief, with apprehension?" But the doctor-narrator
must practice his profession, and so, suppressing his death
anxieties, he goes out to treat his patient. As he does, he

sees his work and all of life in terms of a dance of life and death: "Either dance or annihilation."[37] That night, the patient he is summoned to see will live. The next night, however, he is called to a house where an infant is dying of acute meningitis, and he can do nothing. As this short story ends, we are left with the impression of the ebb and flow of life and death, which the doctor calls the danse pseudo-macabre, as if to make light of his own fears. But the images of the dance and of the doctor as a death-imprinted survivor remain with us, whether or not the author tries to mock—or mask—his apprehensions.

In his first-person narrative "Rounds," Richard Selzer actually describes himself, as well as the widow of one of his patients, as a "survivor." Edna's dying husband is hooked up to all sorts of tubes and life-sustaining gear. Edna wants to kiss her husband but cannot because of all the gear. She asks the surgeon to pull out the tubes; instead, he sends her home to rest.

When Edna returns to the hospital at 8 o'clock that night, her husband's body has already been taken away. The surgeon-narrator describes the scene, highlighting the widow's loss—and his own. "Edna and I sit on opposite sides of the empty bed. Our voices echo. We are hollow-voiced survivors."[38] Obviously, the surgeon feels guilty—guilty that he had sent the wife home (even though he could not have known that her husband would die during those hours); guilty, perhaps, because he had been unable to keep his patient alive; and guilty, probably, because he had prevented the wife from kissing her husband one last time.

> "I'm sorry," [the surgeon says]....
> "You should be," [the wife says].... "You gypped me."[39]

The widow's last words, fired at the surgeon, sting with the survivor's pain and anger. But what the widow-survivor does not realize is that the doctor-survivor is suffering from some of the same emotions she feels: pain, anger, guilt, frustration, and loss.

A doctor, therefore, may be understood as a kind of survivor, as the selections from Gogarty, Williams, and Selzer have illustrated. A doctor may also be portrayed as a survivor by a lay writer, as in Camus's *The Plague*.

THE PLAGUE

Dr. Bernard Rieux, the narrator of Albert Camus's novel *The Plague*, is a survivor in several senses. He is a doctor; he is a person who lives through the plague that closes off his city for months; and he survives not only his close friend, Tarrou, but also his wife. (As the epidemic ends, Dr. Rieux learns that his wife, who had been in a sanitarium out of town, has died of tuberculosis.) Here is the doctor-survivor's story, as Dr. Rieux chronicles it.

Suddenly in "194_," the plague strikes Oran, Algeria, and the city must be quarantined. All the people trapped there become "prisoners of the plague."[40] As time passes, Dr. Rieux finds himself numbed to the pain and suffering around him, and his numbing—which is the survivor's psychic numbing—is his only relief. "Rieux had learned that he need no longer steel himself against pity. One grows out of pity when it's useless. And in this feeling that his heart had slowly closed in on itself, the doctor found a solace, his only solace, for the almost unendurable burden of his days."[41]

As the death toll mounts to nearly seven hundred per week, the doctor and the entire populace suffer from a sense of immersion in death. Because there is no known remedy for the plague, one of the hardest things for Dr. Rieux is that he cannot really help or even try to heal. All he can do is diagnose the disease and then send victims and their families into isolation. And he finds that because he, the doctor, cannot help people, they resent and even hate him.

> Sometimes a woman would clutch his sleeve, crying shrilly: "Doctor, you'll save him, won't you?" But he wasn't there for saving life; he was there to order a sick man's evacuation. How futile was the hatred he saw on faces then! "You haven't

a heart!" a woman told him on one occasion. She was wrong; he had one. It saw him through his twenty-hour day, when he hourly watched men dying who were meant to live. It enabled him to start anew each morning. He had just enough heart for that.[42]

When the weekly death toll finally begins to fall, people start to hope once more. To Rieux, they seem to be "setting forth at last, like a shipload of survivors, toward a land of promise."[43] But the doctor knows that because of their experiences they have been marked by a vision of death they can never erase: "one can't forget everything, however great one's wish to do so; the plague was bound to leave traces . . . in people's hearts."[44]

The doctor, too, is imprinted with death and, therefore, changed forever. Just as the epidemic is slowing down, his friend Tarrou dies. All day and night the doctor sits by his friend's bed, but he is unable to save him: "This human form, his friend's, . . . was foundering under his eyes in the dark flood of the pestilence, and he could do nothing to avert the wreck."[45] The night after Tarrou's death, Rieux has the "feeling that no peace was possible to him henceforth, any more than there can be an armistice for a mother bereaved of her son or for a man who buried his friend."[46]

As the novel ends, Dr. Rieux says that the tale he told of the plague "could not be one of a final victory. It could be only the record of what had had to be done, and what assuredly would have to be done again in the never ending fight . . . by all who . . . strive their utmost to be healers."[47] These words capture something essential about the doctor as a survivor. They suggest that, in one way or another, the doctor is a survivor who strives to be a healer and must continue to strive to be one "in the never ending fight." After all, the struggle against disease and death goes on and on, even though the doctor-survivor knows that in the end he cannot be victorious. But it is the struggle that counts, and it is the continual struggle that continually makes the doctor a survivor, with all the pain and knowledge that that vision implies.

REFLECTIONS

Indelibly marked with the imprint of death, the survivor—whether he is a person who has lived through the horrors of war or some other catastrophe or a doctor who has lived through, and continues to live through, the pain, death, and dying he must face daily as part of his profession—is someone who has learned what it is to fight for life, while knowing that in the end he can never really win. Always, the survivor's eyes are haunted by a vision of death. It is the look of the corpse that gazed back at and never left Elie Wiesel when, for the first time after his ordeal, he looked at himself in a mirror. And it is the look, described by Gogarty's professor of medicine, of always seeing in life "the pull of the grave."

Psychic numbing or "the cessation of feeling," one of the survivor's characteristic traits, as chronicled by Lifton, actually helps explain something essential about a doctor. How often do we hear doctors accused of being cold, unfeeling, or insensitive? But coldness or insensitivity—psychic numbing—is actually a part of the survivor's heritage. And while such numbing is a means to dull pain, it is also a sign of the pain itself, both the survivor's pain and the doctor's pain. There is, after all, no need for this kind of numbing *unless pain is already present.*

We have called the doctor a survivor or a kind of survivor, but by no means do we wish to imply that a doctor is exactly like a survivor who has lived through the magnitude of suffering and death immersion that a survivor of Bataan, Hiroshima, the Nazi death camps, or any other catastrophe has known. The doctor and other survivors share a similarity in kind of experience but not at all in degree. Obviously, while a doctor—like other survivors—knows a death immersion, the intensity of the doctor's experience is totally different because his death immersion does not threaten to engulf him directly or immediately. We think back to Mr. D, the survivor of Bataan. Although he had outlived his terrible past, he was not really able to live or relish life because he had been ruined by what he had survived. And so, when he was dying, he was bitter with his doctor for being, precisely, what he himself had been: a survivor. Yet this unfortunate man who accused his doctor actually had a secret kinship with him which neither the patient nor the physician, at that time, recognized or understood. In fact, this tormented patient helps us understand— and feel—through his muteness, anger, and pain what it means to be a survivor and, in a curiously related way, what it means to be a doctor. Both the patient and the doctor he angrily accused are, in different but related ways, survivors—people whose eyes have been filled with, and forever changed by, an ineradicable image of death.

CONCLUSION

Because so much of the new doctor's experience involves facing death—both the patient's and his own—in various forms (in the cadavers of anatomy class, in patients, in fears), the first three chapters of our book treat different aspects of death.

Chapter 1 explores facing or contemplating death, in general. Starting with the real—but also symbolic—presence of death in the sheet-shrouded corpse being wheeled through the hospital tunnel, we seek to sound the patient's and the physician's silent reactions. Through literature, we examine how several others have faced the prospect, sometimes remote, sometimes imminent, of their own deaths. This chapter ultimately demonstrates that one's attitude toward life is intimately related to one's attitude toward death. Tolstoy's "The Death of Ivan Ilych" and Michie's "A Splendid Day" are particularly poignant examples of this. Contemplating the face of death leads—or should lead—one, eventually, to thinking about life.

Chapter 2 probes the actual physical manifestations of death: the cadaver, rotting corpses, skeletal remains, and so forth. Here is the utter reality of death—its physical aspect and its symbolic import. From the ancient Egyptians who deliberately pursued pleasure while contemplating symbolic corpses to Richard Selzer's detailed depictions of what happens to a corpse, the literary parallels explore the grotesque, real, pitiable, and inevitable end of all men.

Chapter 3 confronts death in a different form: the tragic reality of a twenty-nine-year-old woman's death following childbirth. We were distressed that this woman's doctors had seemed so cold, distant, unemotional, and unhelpful, yet we knew from small signs and from the intern's own feelings that they had actually been distraught. The literary parallels reveal that other doctors behaved in similar ways in similar circumstances. We were able to end this chapter—and this three-chapter section on death—on a high note in the account given by French physician François Mauriceau. For Mauriceau managed to turn the tragedy of his sister's death in childbirth into an inspiration and an impetus for action for his future very successful work in obstetrics.

Turning from the direct contemplation of death, chapters 4 through 7 explore four defenses—ritual, romanticizing, humor, and hatred—that both doctors and patients use, successfully and unsuccessfully, in dealing with suffering, pain, disease, and death. Several times in this work we also write about another very important defense: numbing. All of these defenses help us understand something about doctors and patients.

Chapter 4 introduces ritual, one of the most important elements in the art of medicine. While this chapter focuses on the ritual of the death certificate, which one physician found so calming and healing, that is only one kind of ritual that doctors perform. Although many of a doctor's daily routines have a practical purpose, they also share many elements of ritual. They are repetitive; they *must* be performed in the same, precise way each time; and they serve a purpose—much of it symbolic—that goes far beyond their practical function. For example, the doctor dons a long white coat. The whiteness implies that the coat is clean: this is its practical function. But the white coat is also a symbolic, ritualistic vestment. Think, for instance, of the white vestments that priests wear for Easter Mass in the Roman Catholic Church as a symbol of purity, salvation, and resurrection. At one time, were not doctors, in fact, priests? In Greek temples to Asklepios, god of healing, and in temples to his Roman counterpart, Aesculapius, physician-priests ministered to the sick. The healing divinity Aesculapius was represented by the serpent. The twining serpents of the caduceus—the modern symbol of the medical profession—recall the priestly role of the physician.

Ritual also helps define the doctor-patient relationship, for it provides much of the order and structure through which physicians and patients handle difficult, unpleasant, sometimes unbearable circumstances. Consider, for example, the ritual of morning rounds in the hospital. The doctor puts on his white coat and visits each of his patients each morning. He listens to each patient's lungs and heart, whether that patient is only slightly sick or very ill. The practical purpose is evident: the doctor is ascertaining if his patient's lungs are clear, if his heart is beating normally, and so forth. But the ritual of morning rounds, repeated every day, conveys a symbolic meaning to the patient: he is being cared for, his doctor is checking up on him, not as a chart full of laboratory values but as a human being with lungs and a heart and feelings.

Ritual, therefore, is an essential part of the human medical experience. In practical terms as well as symbolically, it provides an omnipresent support system both for the physician and for the patient.

Romanticizing, a prime form of denial, is another defense used by patients and physicians. Chapter 5 begins with the literary romanticizing of tuberculosis. The case history and analysis illustrate how romanticizing a disease, the doctor's role, and the patient can distort reality. And in this case history, it was the physician who did the romanticizing. Although romanticizing may seem, and sometimes actually is, pleasant, it is really a turning away from reality that may do a disservice to the patient and doctor alike. Yet how many of us, including doctors and patients, have used, and continue to use, romanticizing as a defense?

Chapters 6 and 7 approach elements of medicine that are commonplace in all professions: humor and hatred used as defenses, either positive or negative, for dealing with what is terrible, pathetic, fear inspiring, or outrageous. These chapters also bring out the bond that unites physicians and patients, for at times both doctors and patients resort to the same defenses when thinking about each other or about the problems engendered by illness.

Chapters 8 and 9 return to the open contemplation of death. They describe two patients who did not flee from thoughts of their impending deaths. In fact, the patients in these case histories were successful in accepting their own deaths, not because they used defense or denial, ritual, romanticizing, humor, or hatred but because they savored life and exhibited, even as they were dying, their continuing love of life and other people. These case histories along with the literary parallels depict how death may be approached with dignity, calmness, and even humor. They may, perhaps, serve as models of some of the best answers to the questions about death that were raised in chapters 1 through 7.

Our final chapter, "The Survivor," probes one of the most important aspects of medicine that we have explored: the kinship between the doctor and the patient. Since all physicians—and all people—will know, sooner or later, what the doctor-writer Gogarty called "the pull of the grave," we come to understand how doctors and all people who survive another person's death are, in a sense, absolutely equal. Only time and space separate the survivor from the person who has just died—the doctor from his patient, a grieving relative or friend from a person he has just lost. It would be good if an understanding of this kinship between the patient and the physician could be used to cement a closer understanding and love between them.

We have tried to explore what is means to be a doctor and what it means to be a patient; that is, what it means to be a human being who must face pain and suffering, despair and hope, hate and love, anger and courage, wounds and healing, death and life. We know, of course, that our book is but a small beginning. What is really needed by physicians, other health care professionals, patients, and potential patients—people, in other words—is a broad, lifetime commitment to the human. We are all, as the poet Villon said, "human brothers." We hope that these chapters in a young physician's life, the literary parallels, and our combined reflections will inspire the reader to see, and to seek in great literature, a means to deepen his understanding of the human experience of medicine. For medical life, as we see it, is human life at its most intense. And essentially medicine is—or should be—a human experience.

NOTES

PREFACE

1. Enid Rhodes Peschel, ed., *Medicine and Literature* (New York: Neale Watson Academic Publications, 1980).

INTRODUCTION

1. Edmund D. Pellegrino, "Introduction," in *Medicine and Literature,* p. xvii.
2. Virginia Woolf, "How It Strikes a Contemporary," in *The Common Reader,* p. 302.

1: THE FACE OF DEATH

1. Sophocles, *Antigone,* pp. 135–136.
2. William Shakespeare, *Measure for Measure,* Act III, sc. 1, lines 11–13, p. 1014.
3. Michel de Montaigne, "That to Philosophize is to Learn to Die," in *The Complete Essays of Montaigne,* Bk. I, chap. 20, pp. 56–60.

4. Ibid., p. 59.   5. Ibid., Bk. II, chap. 7, pp. 575–576.
6. Ibid., p. 578.   7. Ibid., p. 576.
8. Ibid., "On the Education of Children," Bk. I, chap. 26, p. 120.
9. Montaigne, *The Complete Works of Montaigne*, p. 1018.
10. Montaigne, *The Complete Essays of Montaigne*, Bk. III, chap. 13, p. 853.
11. Ibid., Bk. III, chap. 12, p. 805.
12. Leo Tolstoy, "The Death of Ivan Ilych," in *Death in Literature*, p. 394.
13. Ibid., p. 409.   14. Ibid.   15. Ibid., p. 410.
16. Ibid., pp. 415–416.   17. Ibid., p. 418.
18. Ibid., pp. 419–420.   19. Ibid., p. 423.
20. Ibid., p. 424.   21. Ibid., p. 433.
22. Ibid., pp. 436–437.   23. Ibid., p. 438.
24. Ibid., pp. 437–438.   25. Ibid., p. 439.
26. Ibid., p. 440.
27. William Butler Yeats, "An Irish Airman Foresees his Death," in *Selected Poems and Two Plays of William Butler Yeats*, p. 55.
28. André Malraux, *La Condition humaine*, p. 259. English translations are by Enid Rhodes Peschel.
29. Ibid., p. 260.
30. Ibid., p. 261.
31. Ibid., p. 262.
32. Michael Casey, *Obscenities*, p. 53.
33. Ibid., p. 26.
34. Alexander Solzhenitsyn, *Cancer Ward*, p. 449.
35. Ibid., p. 450.   36. Ibid.   37. Ibid., p. 454.
38. Ibid., p. 458.
39. Molly Ingle Michie, "A Splendid Day," *Virginia Quarterly Review*, p. 412.
40. Ibid., p. 410.   41. Ibid., p. 411.
42. Ibid., p. 415.
43. Ibid., pp. 413–414.
44. Ibid., p. 414.
45. Ibid., p. 421.
46. Ibid., pp. 422–423.
47. Charles Baudelaire, "The Clock," in *Four French Symbolist Poets*, p. 137.

2: MY CADAVER

1. Herodotus, *The History of Herodotus*, pp. 64–65.
2. Edward F. Chaney, *François Villon in His Environment*, p. 25.
3. J. Huizinga, *Le Déclin du moyen âge*, p. 167. English translations are by Enid Rhodes Peschel.
4. Carla Gottlieb, "Modern Art and Death," in *The Meaning of Death*, p. 160.
5. Huizinga, p. 173.
6. James M. Clark, *The Dance of Death in the Middle Ages and the Renaissance*, p. 27.
7. Ibid.   8. Ibid., p. 22.
9. Chaney, p. 59.
10. Clark, p. 24.
11. Huizinga, p. 178.
12. Chaney, p. 46.
13. François Villon, *Testament*, XLI, in *The Complete Works of François Villon*, p. 38. Translated by Enid Rhodes Peschel.
14. Villon, "L'Épitaphe Villon (Ballade des pendus)" in *The Complete Works*, p. 162. Translated by Enid Rhodes Peschel.
15. Donald Frame, *François Rabelais*, p. 5.
16. Marc Chassaigne, *Étienne Dolet*, p. 129.
17. Frame, p. 17.
18. Joseph Boulmier, *Estienne Dolet*, p. 198. Translations are by Enid Rhodes Peschel.
19. François Rabelais, *The Histories of Gargantua and Pantagruel*, Bk. I, chap. 27, pp. 99–100.
20. Ibid., Bk. II, chap. 3, p. 177. J. M. Cohen, the translator of the English edition we quote, uses "coney" (instead of "cunt") for the French *con*.
21. Gottfried Benn, "Man and Woman Go through the Cancer Ward," in *Primal Vision: Selected Writings of Gottfried Benn*, p. 217.
22. Richard Selzer, "The Corpse," in *Mortal Lessons*, p. 130.
23. Ibid., pp. 131–132.   24. Ibid., pp. 134–135.
25. Ibid., pp. 136–137.   26. Ibid., p. 140.
27. Rabelais, Bk. I, chap. 5, p. 182.

3: "BUT WHAT IF SHE SHOULD DIE?"

1. Leo Tolstoy, *War and Peace,* p. 351.
2. Ibid., p. 352.   3. Ibid., p. 353.   4. Ibid.
5. Ibid., pp. 353–354.   6. Ibid., p. 354.
7. Ernest Hemingway, *A Farewell to Arms,* pp. 320–321.
8. Ibid., p. 322.   9. Ibid., p. 325.
10. Ibid., pp. 329–330.   11. Ibid., p. 330.
12. Ibid., p. 331.   13. Ibid., pp. 331–332.
14. Ibid., p. 332.
15. W. Somerset Maugham, *A Summing Up,* p. 17.
16. W. Somerset Maugham, *Liza of Lambeth,* p. 8.
17. Ibid., p. 116–117.   18. Ibid., p. 118.
19. Ibid., pp. 119–120.   20. Ibid., p. 120.
21. Ibid., p. 121.   22. Ibid., p. 123.   23. Ibid.
24. Ibid., p. 125.   25. Ibid.
26. Harold Speert, M.D., *Obstetric and Gynecological Milestones,* p. 564.
27. François Mauriceau, *Traité des maladies des femmes grosses et de celles qui sont accouchées,* p. 162. All translations of Mauriceau are by Enid Rhodes Peschel.
28. Ibid., p. 163.   29. Ibid., p. 166.
30. Ibid., p. 168.

4: RITUAL AND THE DEATH CERTIFICATE

1. Jurgen Ludwig, M.D., "Editorial," in *Mayo Clinic Proceedings,* p. 347.
2. Ibid.
3. George C. Homans, "Anxiety and Ritual," in *Reader in Comparative Religion,* p. 117.
4. Clyde Kluckhohn, "Myths and Rituals," in *Reader in Comparative Religion,* p. 141.
5. Ibid., p. 146.
6. William Blake, "The Divine Image," in *Poetry and Prose of William Blake,* p. 58.
7. Kahlil Gibran, *The Prophet,* p. 67.
8. John Carey, *John Donne,* p. 136.

9. John Donne, *Devotions upon Emergent Occasions*, pp. 107–109.
10. Ibid., pp. 112–113.
11. John Donne, "Oh, to vex me, contraries meet in one . . . ," in *The Oxford Anthology of English Literature*, Vol. I, pp. 1052–1053.
12. Homans, "Anxiety and Ritual," p. 117.
13. Ibid.

5: THE FALLEN WOMAN

1. René Dubos and Jean Dubos, *The White Plague*, p. 10.
2. In ibid., p. 9.   3. Ibid., p. 11.   4. Ibid., p. 14.
5. Ibid., p. 84.
6. Harrison's *Principles of Internal Medicine*, p. 858.
7. William Cullen Bryant, *Poetical Works of William Cullen Bryant*, p. 54.
8. Giuseppe Verdi, *La Traviata*, p. 8. All translations of *La Traviata* are by Enid Rhodes Peschel.
9. Ibid., pp. 96–97.   10. Ibid., pp. 102–103.
11. Ibid., pp. 104–106.   12. Ibid., pp. 143–146.
13. Ibid., pp. 149–150.   14. Ibid., p. 150.
15. Ibid., pp. 151–154.   16. Ibid., pp. 154–156.
17. Ibid., pp. 164–170.   18. Ibid., pp. 180–181.
19. Ibid., p. 246.   20. Ibid., pp. 289–319.
21. Ibid., p. 325.   22. Ibid., pp. 330–333.
23. Ibid., pp. 350–358.   24. Ibid., pp. 363–364.
25. Ibid., p. 375.   26. Ibid., pp. 378–380.
27. Ibid., pp. 380–381.   28. Ibid., pp. 383–385.

6: ABERRANT MEDICAL HUMOR

1. Renée Fox, *Experiment Perilous*, esp. pp. 75–82, 246, 253.
2. François Rabelais, *Gargantua and Pantagruel*, Bk. I, chap. 35, p. 116.

3. In William Carlos Williams, *The Farmers' Daughters*, pp. 158–166.
4. In Richard Selzer, *Mortal Lessons*, pp. 62–77.
5. William B. Ober, "Can the Leper Change His Spots?" *American Journal of Dermatopathology*, pp. 43–58, 173–186.
6. Fox, pp. 81, 253–254.
7. Leo Tolstoy, *War and Peace*, p. 884.
8. Ibid., p. 886.   9. Ibid.
10. Mark Harris, *Something about a Soldier*, p. 119.
11. James Jones, *The Thin Red Line*, p. 53.
12. Ibid., pp. 69–71.
13. Erich Maria Remarque, *All Quiet on the Western Front*, pp. 9–10.
14. Ibid., pp. 125, 202.   15. Ibid., p. 124.
16. William Shakespeare, *Cymbeline*, Act V, sc. 5, ll. 29–30, p. 1276.
17. Remarque, p. 115.
18. William Shakespeare, *Hamlet*, Act V, sc. 1, ll. 38–66, 108–125, pp. 536–541.
19. Sigmund Freud, "Jokes and Their Relation to the Unconscious," p. 229.
20. Ibid., p. 230.
21. Fox, p. 60.
22. Ibid., p. 175.
23. In Fox, p. 175.
24. William Blake, "The Marriage of Heaven and Hell," in *Poetry and Prose of William Blake*, p. 184.
25. Mark Van Doren, "Wit," in *Collected Poems*, p. 241.

7: WHEN A DOCTOR HATES A PATIENT

1. William Carlos Williams, *The Autobiography of William Carlos Williams*, p. 286.
2. Ibid., p. 93.   3. Ibid., p. 95.
4. William Carlos Williams, "The Use of Force," in *The Farmers' Daughters*, p. 131.
5. Ibid., p. 133.   6. Ibid., p. 134.   7. Ibid.

8. Ibid., p. 135.   9. Ibid.
10. Richard Selzer, "Brute," in *Letters to a Young Doctor,* p. 60.
11. Ibid.   12. Ibid., p. 61.   13. Ibid.
14. Ibid., p. 62.   15. Ibid.
16. Ibid., p. 63.

8: SOME LESSONS FROM THE CANCER WARD

1. Letter from Leonard DiLisio, Assistant to Mr. Solzhenitsyn, dated August 20, 1982, Cavendish, Vermont, to Enid Rhodes Peschel.
2. Solzhenitsyn, *Cancer Ward,* p. 1.
3. Ibid., p. 3.   4. Ibid., p. 2.   5. Ibid., p. 7.
6. Ibid., p. 10.   7. Ibid.   8. Ibid., p. 16.
9. Because of her interest in Kostoglotov, Dr. Vera Gangart decides to read every scientific paper "that described how hormone therapy should be used to combat seminoma" (*Cancer Ward,* p. 343).
10. Solzhenitsyn, *Cancer Ward,* pp. 63–64.
11. Ibid., p. 153.   12. Ibid., p. 80.   13. Ibid., p. 82.
14. Ibid., p. 460.   15. Ibid., p. 489.
16. Ibid., p. 488.   17. Ibid., pp. 492–493.
18. Ibid., p. 496.   19. Ibid., pp. 524–525.
20. Ibid., p. 532.
21. Seneca, *The Morals of Seneca,* p. 137.
22. Montaigne, "Of Experience," in *The Complete Essays of Montaigne,* p. 837.

9: "AM I IN HEAVEN NOW?"

1. Emily Dickinson, #764, in *The Complete Poems of Emily Dickinson,* p. 374.
2. Ivan Turgenev, "Death," in *The Novels of Ivan Turgenev: A Sportsman's Sketches,* pp. 30–32.
3. Ibid., p. 38.

4. Richard B. Sewall, *The Life of Emily Dickinson*, p. 530.
5. Dickinson, #214, in *The Complete Poems of Emily Dickinson*, pp. 98–99.
6. Ibid., #280, pp. 128–129.   7. Ibid., #692, p. 341.
8. Ibid., #1052, p. 480.   9. Ibid., #1544, p. 644.
10. Ibid., #1558, p. 648.
11. Ibid., #324, pp. 153–154.

10: THE SURVIVOR

1. Donald Knox, *Death March*, pp. 119, 155.
2. Ibid., p. 134.   3. Ibid., p. 150.   4. Ibid., p. 165.
5. Ibid., p. 166.   6. Ibid., p. 202.
7. Ibid., p. 209.   8. Ibid., pp. 338–347.
9. Ibid., p. 350.   10. Ibid.   11. Ibid., p. 378.
12. Ibid., pp. 461–462.   13. Ibid., pp. 462–463.
14. Ibid., pp. 478–479.   15. Ibid., p. 475.
16. Ibid., pp. 475–476.
17. Robert Jay Lifton, *Death in Life*, pp. 479–480.
18. Ibid., pp. 10, 6.   19. Ibid., p. 481.
20. Ibid., p. 496.   21. Ibid., p. 34.
22. Ibid., p. 35.   23. Ibid., pp. 483–484.
24. Ibid., p. 500.   25. Ibid., p. 34.
26. Ibid., p. 504.
27. Elie Wiesel, *Night*, p. 32.
28. Ibid., p. 101.   29. Ibid., p. 106.
30. Ibid., p. 109.
31. Elie Wiesel, *The Accident*, p. 4.
32. Ibid., pp. 52–53.   33. Ibid., p. 76.
34. Oliver St. John Gogarty, *Tumbling in the Hay*, pp. 245–247.
35. William Carlos Williams, "The Visit," in *The Selected Poems of William Carlos Williams*, p. 117.
36. William Carlos Williams, "Danse Pseudomacabre," in *The Farmers' Daughters*, p. 208.
37. Ibid., p. 210.
38. Richard Selzer, "Rounds," in *Letters to a Young Doctor*, p. 91.

39. Ibid.
40. Albert Camus, *The Plague,* p. 66.
41. Ibid., p. 86.   42. Ibid., p. 178.   43. Ibid., p. 254.
44. Ibid., p. 259.   45. Ibid., pp. 268–269.
46. Ibid., p. 269.   47. Ibid., p. 287.

BIBLIOGRAPHY OF WORKS QUOTED

Baudelaire, Charles. "The Clock." In *Four French Symbolist Poets: Baudelaire, Rimbaud, Verlaine, Mallarmé.* Translation and Introduction by Enid Rhodes Peschel. Athens: Ohio University Press, 1981.

Benn, Gottfried. "Man and Woman Go through the Cancer Ward." Translated by Babette Deutsch. In *Primal Vision: Selected Writings of Gottfried Benn.* Edited by E. B. Ashton. New York: New Directions, 1971.

Blake, William. *Poetry and Prose of William Blake.* Edited by Geoffrey Keynes. London: The Nonesuch Library, 1961.

Boulmier, Joseph. *Estienne Dolet: Sa Vie, ses oeuvres, son martyr.* Paris: August Aubry, 1857.

Bryant, William Cullen. *Poetical Works of William Cullen Bryant.* New York: Appleton and Co., 1901.

Camus, Albert. *The Plague.* Translated by Stuart Gilbert. New York: Vintage Books, 1972.

Carey, John. *John Donne: Life, Mind and Art.* New York: Oxford University Press, 1981.

Casey, Michael. *Obscenities.* New Haven and London: Yale University Press, 1972.

Chaney, Edward F. *François Villon in His Environment.* Oxford: B. H. Blackwell, Ltd., 1946.

Chassaigne, Marc. *Étienne Dolet: Portraits et documents inédits.* Paris: Albin Michel, Éditeur, 1930.

Clark, James M. *The Dance of Death in the Middle Ages and the Renaissance.* Glasgow: Jackson, Son & Company, 1950.

Dickinson, Emily. *The Complete Poems of Emily Dickinson.* Edited by Thomas H. Johnson. Boston and Toronto: Little, Brown and Company, 1960.

Donne, John. "Oh, to vex me, contraries meet in one . . . " In *The Oxford Anthology of English Literature* Vol. I. Edited by Frank Kermode and John Hollander. New York, London, Toronto: Oxford University Press, 1973.

—————. *Devotions upon Emergent Occasions.* Ann Arbor: The University of Michigan Press, 1975.

Dubos, René, and Jean Dubos. *The White Plague: Tuberculosis, Man and Society.* Boston: Little, Brown and Company, 1952.

Fox, Renée. *Experiment Perilous: Physicians and Patients Facing the Unknown.* Glencoe, Ill.: The Free Press, 1959.

Frame, Donald. *François Rabelais: A Study.* New York and London: Harcourt Brace Jovanovich, 1977.

Freud, Sigmund. "Jokes and Their Relation to the Unconscious." In *The Standard Edition of the Complete Psychological Works of Sigmund Freud.* Vol. 8. Translator and General Editor, James Strachey. London: Hogarth Press, 1974.

Gogarty, Oliver St. John. *Tumbling in the Hay.* London: Constable and Company, Ltd., 1939.

Gottlieb, Carla. "Modern Art and Death." In *The Meaning of Death.* Edited by Herman Feifel. New York, London, Sydney, Toronto: McGraw-Hill Book Company, 1959. Pp. 157–188.

Harris, Mark. *Something about a Soldier.* New York: The Macmillan Company, 1957.

Harrison's *Principles of Internal Medicine.* 7th ed. New York: McGraw-Hill, Inc., 1974.

Hemingway, Ernest. *A Farewell to Arms.* New York: Charles Scribner's Sons, 1929. Renewed copyright 1957 by Ernest Hemingway.

Herodotus. *The History of Herodotus.* In *Great Books of the Western World.* Vol. 6. Edited by Robert Maynard Hutchins.

Chicago, London, Toronto: Encyclopaedia Britannica, Inc., 1952.

Homans, George C. "Anxiety and Ritual: The Theories of Malinowski and Radcliffe-Brown." In *Reader in Comparative Religion: An Anthropological Approach.* Edited by William A. Lessa and Evon Z. Vogt. Evanston, Ill., and White Plains, N.Y.: Row, Peterson and Company, 1958. Pp. 112–118.

Huizinga, J. *Le Déclin du moyen âge.* Paris: Payot, 1961.

Jones, James. *The Thin Red Line.* New York: Charles Scribner's Sons, 1962.

Kluckhohn, Clyde. "Myths and Rituals: A General Theory." In *Reader in Comparative Religion: An Anthropological Approach.* Edited by William A. Lessa and Evon Z. Vogt. Evanston, Ill., and White Plains, N.Y.: Row, Peterson and Company, 1958. Pp. 135–151.

Knox, Donald. *Death March: The Survivors of Bataan.* New York and London: Harcourt Brace Jovanovich, 1981.

Lifton, Robert Jay. *Death in Life: Survivors of Hiroshima.* New York: Basic Books, Inc., 1967.

Ludwig, Jurgen, M.D. "Editorial." *Mayo Clinic Proceedings* 55, 5 (May 1980), 347–348.

Malraux, André. *La Condition humaine.* Paris: Gallimard, 1946.

Maugham, W. Somerset. *A Summing Up.* New York: Doubleday, Doran & Company, Inc., 1938.

———. *Liza of Lambeth.* Harmondsworth: Penguin Books, 1967. Reprint 1978.

Mauriceau, François. *Traité des maladies des femmes grosses et de celles qui sont accouchées.* Vol. I. 6th ed. Paris: Par la Compagnie des Libraires, 1721.

Michie, Molly Ingle. "A Splendid Day." *Virginia Quarterly Review* 56, 3 (Summer 1980), 410–423.

Montaigne, Michel de. *The Complete Works of Montaigne: Essays, Travel Journal, Letters.* Translated by Donald M. Frame. Stanford: Stanford University Press, 1957.

———. *The Complete Essays of Montaigne.* Translated by Donald M. Frame. Stanford: Stanford University Press, 1958.

Ober, William B. "Can the Leper Change His Spots?" *American Journal of Dermatopathology* 5, 1 and 2 (Feb. 1983 and April 1983), 43–58, 173–186.

Pellegrino, Edmund D. "Introduction: To Look Feelingly—The Affinities of Medicine and Literature." In *Medicine and Literature.* Edited by Enid Rhodes Peschel. New York: Neale Watson Academic Publications, 1980. Pp. xv–xix.

Peschel, Enid Rhodes, ed. *Medicine and Literature.* New York: Neale Watson Academic Publications, 1980.

Rabelais, François. *The Histories of Gargantua and Pantagruel.* Translated by J. M. Cohen. Baltimore: Penguin Books, 1963.

Remarque, Erich Maria. *All Quiet on the Western Front.* Translated by A. W. Wheen. New York: Fawcett Crest, 1975.

Selzer, Richard. *Mortal Lessons: Notes on the Art of Surgery.* New York: Simon and Schuster, 1976.

————. *Letters to a Young Doctor.* New York: Simon and Schuster, 1982.

Seneca. *The Morals of Seneca: A Selection of his Prose.* Edited by Walter Clode. London: Walter Scott, 1888.

Sewall, Richard B. *The Life of Emily Dickinson.* New York: Farrar, Straus and Giroux, 1980.

Shakespeare, William. *Cymbeline.* In *The London Shakespeare.* Vol. II. Edited by John Munro. New York: Simon and Schuster, 1957. Pp. 1176–1291.

————. *Hamlet.* In *The London Shakespeare.* Vol. V. Edited by John Munro. New York: Simon and Schuster, 1957. Pp. 371–571.

————. *Measure for Measure.* In *The London Shakespeare.* Vol. II. Edited by John Munro. New York: Simon and Schuster, 1957. Pp. 975–1066.

Solzhenitsyn, Alexander. *Cancer Ward.* Translated by Nicholas Bethell and David Burg. New York: Farrar, Straus and Giroux, 1974.

Sophocles. *Antigone.* In *The Theban Plays.* Translated by E. F. Watling. Baltimore: Penguin Books, 1947. Reprint 1962.

Speert, Harold, M.D. *Obstetric and Gynecologic Milestones: Essays in Eponymy.* New York: The Macmillan Company, 1958.

Tolstoy, Leo. *War and Peace.* Translated by Louise and Aylmer Maude. New York: Simon and Schuster, 1942.

————. "The Death of Ivan Ilych." In *Death in Literature.* Edited by Robert F. Weir. New York: Columbia University Press, 1980. Pp. 386–440.

Turgenev, Ivan. *The Novels of Ivan Turgenev: A Sportsman's Sketches*. Vol. II. Translated by Constance Garnett. New York: The Macmillan Company; London: William Heinemann, 1920.

Van Doren, Mark. "Wit." In *Collected Poems: 1922–1938*. New York: Henry Holt and Company, 1939.

Verdi, Giuseppe. *La Traviata*. Libretto by Francesco Maria Piave. Milan: G. Ricordi & Company, 1962.

Villon, François. *The Complete Works of François Villon*. New York: Bantam Books, 1960.

Wiesel, Elie. *The Accident*. Translated by Anne Borchardt. Toronto, New York, London, Sydney: Bantam Books, 1982.

_____. *Night*. Translated by Stella Rodway. Toronto, New York, London, Sydney: Bantam Books, 1982.

Williams, William Carlos. *The Autobiography of William Carlos Williams*. New York: New Directions, 1951.

_____. *The Farmers' Daughters: The Collected Stories of William Carlos Williams*. New York: New Directions, 1961.

_____. *The Selected Poems of William Carlos Williams*. New York: New Directions, 1969.

Woolf, Virginia. "How It Strikes a Contemporary." In *The Common Reader*. London: The Hogarth Press, 1925.

Yeats, William Butler. "An Irish Airman Foresees his Death." In *Selected Poems and Two Plays of William Butler Yeats*. Edited by M. L. Rosenthal. New York: The Macmillan Company, 1962.

Designer: Cheryl Carrington
Compositor: Auto-Graphics, Inc.
Text: 11/13 Cheltenham
Display: Cheltenham

Lightning Source UK Ltd.
Milton Keynes UK
UKHW012121110222
398568UK00001B/13